Chronic Total Occlusion

After the Heart Attack,
the Statins
and Restenosis

Mike Stone

Chronic Total Occlusion is intended solely for informational purposes and is not intended as personal medical advice. Personal medical advice should be obtained from your own doctor or other qualified medical authority.

Chronic Total Occlusion supersedes *The Next 20,*000 first published in 2007, which is no longer available.

Heart Recovery Publishing
2028 Sawmill Road
River Ridge, La 70123

ISBN 978-1-451-59424-9

Library of Congress Control Number: 2010904639

Cover design by the author
    Front cover original photograph:
    http://www.heartrecovery.net/pictures.html
    Cross Golan bike trip April 3-4, 2009
    Golan Heights, Israel
    Heart borrowed from *Surviving a Successful Heart Attack*

To Esty and the kids-
Naamah, Sagi, Rakefet and Tuval

Back Cover

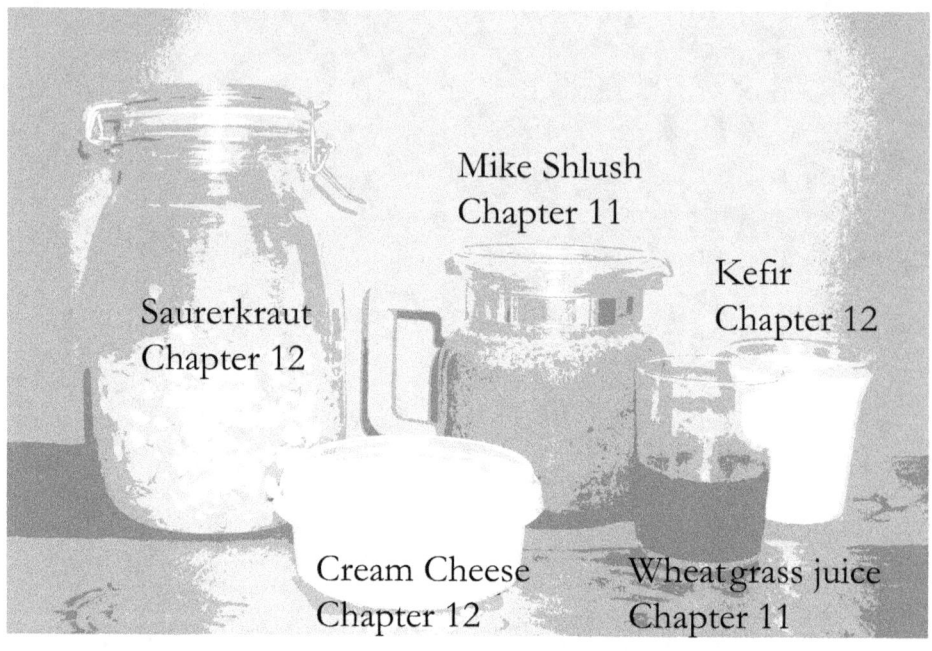

Saurerkraut
Chapter 12

Mike Shlush
Chapter 11

Kefir
Chapter 12

Cream Cheese
Chapter 12

Wheatgrass juice
Chapter 11

Yes, this is the actual color of my kitchen wall.

Arms and Hands Acknowledgements

Tuval – page 32, page 127
Limor – page 128

Contents

	Author's Note	vi
	Preface	x
1	What Kind of Name is that for a Book?	1
2	What Really Worries Me	4
3	Uh-Oh – What's Wrong?	9
4	Raw Food & Enzymes	14
5	Why is Raw Food so Unappealing?	29
6	Pasteur – Hero or Villain?	36
7	Post Pasteur	47
8	Two Postulates	62
9	A Very Thin Chapter on Fats	66
10	What's New Since SASHA?	76
11	Green Gold	102
12	Fermenting	117
13	Aw Nuts	133
14	The Next 20,000	139
15	What Really are Degenerative Diseases?	155
16	Angiogram #2	161
17	Vindication	165
18	Bottom Line	171
19	Epilogue	191
20	Post-Epilogue	199
21	2010	202
	References	205

Author's Note

Chronic Total Occlusion is an updated version of *The Next 20,000* which was first published in 2007 and essentially supersedes it. With this publication, *The Next 20,000* will no longer be available. Besides a face lift, formatting changes and minor changes throughout, the main changes are significant updates to Chapter 18 (my ever changing and improving daily eating habits) and the addition of chapter 21. In Chapter 21, I introduce a new concept - 'Post Statin Syndrome'.

It was not my intention to rewrite and thoroughly revise *The Next 20,000*. For instance, in Chapter 10, I discuss new technologies and reference 20 different research papers published between 2006 and 2007 regarding the pleiotropic (cholesterol-independent) effects of statins. There was no point in reinforcing these findings with more of the same type research papers from 2009.

The Next 20,000, and now *Chronic Total Occlusion*, is the natural sequel to my *Surviving a Successful Heart Attack* first published in 2004 and later revised and distributed via the national networks in 2005. From hereafter, any reference to *Surviving a Successful Heart Attack* will be according to its initials SASHA. SASHA was written during a much more naive stage of my life. The term 'statin' and its true significance entered into my vocabulary only several years after my heart attack, as did the real significance of the term 'cholesterol'. What do I mean by naivety? In SASHA I stated

> *Again, it is not my purpose to medically judge which side is valid. It is my purpose to state that*

many of the self-evident truths regarding health
and nutrition that we have grown up believing to
be absolute, may not be true!

'May not be true' is fitting for someone sitting on the fence, not knowing for sure which way to decide. *Chronic Total Occlusion* starts out under the premise that cholesterol and saturated fat are not the causes of heart disease.* Period. End of story. Correlation, when occurring, does not indicate causation. All my life I have driven manual transmission vehicles. Several months before my heart attack in 2001, I started driving an automatic transmission car. Does that make automatic transmissions a risk factor for heart disease?

Anyone still needing further clarification regarding this subject should read the classic *The Cholesterol Myths* by Dr. Uffe Ravnskov and/or the more recent *The Great Cholesterol Con* by Anthony Colpo.

I had two main purposes when deciding to write this book. The first was to let the readers of SASHA know what has become of Mike and his stent after discontinuing the statins and recovering from the two difficult, statin-induced side-effect years. The second purpose of this book was to give a living example that it is possible to adapt to what may be conceived as unconventional health habits while still living in a conventional household.

Growing and juicing wheatgrass, preparing a daily glass of naturally fermented kefir and even cheese making are not rituals that can only be accomplished by the die-hard naturalist health freaks. They are not that difficult to

---

* The premise that heart disease is caused by high cholesterol levels in the blood is known as the lipid (blood) hypothesis. This term will appear throughout the book.

do and can be integrated into normal routines and normal households.

Does that mean that all other family members have adopted my new habits? Unfortunately not. For most people, status quo evolves from an environment that one was born into. If I could turn back the clock 25 years, there are many things I would have done differently in raising the kids. I would have made English the language of the household. I would have also introduced them to my present eating habits from age 0. I guess that's what the Almighty invented grandkids for (when the eventually time comes).

This book is not a medical reference book in the classic sense. I am not medically trained. That said, I have recommended specific references throughout this book for people who do want further information from reliable sources.

Acknowledgements corner:

I am again indebted to Garry Borsi for his constant source of information and inspiration.

Thanks to Al Brandler for his assistance with the research.

Thanks to Tony Wiseman and Orit Josefi Wiseman of the Outlook Organization, for doing what they do.........

I greatly appreciate the unbound patience of our family physician Dr. Ayala Laufer.

I am also indebted to many individuals whom I have never met personally for the courtesy and time they took from busy schedules to personally answer the frequent questions I had regarding their published works. They really do care.

This list includes (in alphabetical order): Prof. Wilhelm Bloch, Mr. Anthony Colpo, Prof. John P. Cooke, Dr. Ron Grisanti, Dr. Duane Graveline, Prof. Jan Hoff, Dr. Joel Kauffman, Dr. Katharina Meyer, Dr. Ho-Jin Park, Prof Wolfgang Schaper, Dr. Ron Schmid, Prof. Ronald L Terjung, Prof. Axel Urhausen and Prof. Steve H.T. Yang.

Ultimately, the personal habits I have adopted over the last several years are of my own choosing and responsibility. They are not necessarily consistent with all the opinions of the fine people aforementioned, not in their published works nor in personal correspondence with me.

And of course, and foremost, a big hug and kiss to Esty who *still* puts up with me…… and to Naamah, Sagi, Rakefet and Tuval, who wound up with a dad that does things a little bit differently.

Mike Stone
July, 2007, *The Next 20,000*
March, 2010, *Chronic Total Occlusion*

Preface

From the back cover: Pick the one that's different from the others

Fereydoon Batmanghelidj   Ron Grisanti
Victoria Boutenko   Kilmer McCully
Anthony Colpo   Stephen Joseph
William Douglass II   Uffe Ravnskov
Mary Enig   Howard Roark
Sally Fallon Morell   Ron Schmid
Duane Graveline   Anne Wigmore

What do they all have in common?

How did you manage with the questionnaire on the back cover? The correct answer is Howard Roark. Howard Roark was a fictional character; he was the hero in Ayn Rand's epic *The Fountainhead*. He was an architect by profession and refused to lower his standards and accept the consensus ad hoc. As a result, he paid a heavy price in his personal and professional life.

The others are/were real-life personalities. They all promote health and dietary doctrines often conflicting with governmental health regulatory agencies, and ultimately the consensus accepted by the public at large. Some of them have also paid a heavy personal/professional price for advocating their beliefs.

Howard Roark was simply a fictional architect. He was not concerned about his fasting glucose level or the amount of trans-fat in his diet.

There is, however, a bit of Howard Roark in all of them.

The cure is secondary;
the key is prevention.

What Kind of Name is that for a Book?

*What signifies knowing the Names, if you
know not the Natures of things.*
Benjamin Franklin[1]

The previous version of this book was titled *The Next 20,000*. What kind of name is that for a book, especially a book regarding life after a heart attack? This particular name has special personal significance for me. Those who have read SASHA can probably make an educated guess as to what the 20,000 represents. During the writing of this book, this significance changed somewhat even for me, as will be discussed later on.

A better name and one with Internet Search Engine Optimization significance could be something like 'How to Beat Heart Disease' assuming it hasn't already been taken. But no, this really is not a fitting title for a book authored by me simply because I am not a doctor, nor do I have any accredited medical training. This might be a fitting title if authored by Dr. Christiaan Barnard, who performed the world's first heart transplant in Cape Town, South Africa in 1967.

Let me change this example around somewhat. If you were looking for a classy book about rebuilding your carburetor, would you buy a book called 'Overhauling Your Carburetor' by Dr. Christiaan Bernard, Heart Surgeon? Probably not. However, if the book was called 'Overhauling Your Carburetor' by John DeLorean, the developer of the original Pontiac GTO in the sixties, and the DeLorean car that starred in *Back to the Future* in the eighties, you just might buy it. So what if he was later arrested for drug trafficking -- he definitely knew his carburetors!

A better name yet, a name that I would be entitled to use, could be 'How I Beat Heart Disease'. Let's analyze this name for a moment. I had my heart attack at age 51 and discontinued the statins at age 53. If I succeed in living to the ripe old age of 93 without the statins, then no doubt I will have certainly earned the right to use that name. However, if I continue to lead a full life and make it to only 83 years old, what then? Yes, 83 is still considered to be a ripe old age, which would be 30 statin-less years. So again, I will have earned the right to use this title.

Let's take off another ten years. What if I lead a full life without the statin side effects until the age of 73? Now we are getting to a judgment call. Seventy-three is not considered to be especially old these days. How does one compare 20 years of full, no statin side effect years to 30 or more years of simple human existence without the ability to experience all that life has to offer? This is assuming of course that the statins would keep me alive longer as

2

present cardiology guidelines dictate. And finally, if I only make it to 63, that is ten years of living and experiencing life as compared to possibly a couple of decades more of simple existence. Now that's a real tough call!

No, it is still much too early to pick 'How I Beat Heart Disease' for a title. At the time, I decided to stay with *The Next 20,000*.

2

What Really Worries Me

*About half the men and women under sixty-five who have
had a heart attack die within eight years
of the precipitating event.*
Dr. Louis J. Ignarro[2], Nobel Prize 1998 (medicine)

Statistics can be very misleading. Dr. Uffe Ravnskov proved this by his analysis of many research studies claiming to give legitimacy to the lipid hypothesis. The significance of results interpreted according to relative risks as opposed to absolute risks is very misleading and contradictory.[3]

Stats may be useful for analyzing the macro; however, they can be misleading at the micro level. Air travel is still statistically the safest way to travel. For anyone having the misfortune of being on one of those relatively few planes that do crash, his/her loss is a full 100%.

The chances of being killed due to a plane hitting a building you happen to be in approach zero. There are

4

approximately 6.6 billion people in the world today. You figure out the odds of this happening. All lotteries offer you better odds than that, and when was the last time you won a major lottery? For those unfortunate 3,000 or so innocent victims killed on 9/11, the statistics are worthless.

Once a year, I have my annual outpatient rendezvous with the dedicated professor of cardiology who personally supervised my 'heart attack week'.[4] I come to the hospital prepared with the results of my blood tests taken at my local health clinic; I also bring the results of a recent (annual) stress test performed at the hospital associated with my health clinic.

The first order of business after presenting the nurse on duty with all the proper documentation from my health clinic is to undergo an immediate electrocardiogram. When my turn comes to enter his office, he is already reviewing his history notes in my patient file. The first entries were obviously all the events of the eight days of hospitalization in July, 2001, followed by my performance at his rehabilitation course I did at the hospital. He then goes over the original semi-annual monitoring of my condition, which has since been downgraded to an annual visit.

Over the last couple of annual visits, the dialogue starts the same.

"I have a problem with you," he opens.

"I know," is my reply.

"According to these cholesterol results you should go back on the statins."

The next few minutes are spent on his attempts to convince me to return to a statin, or as an alternative, at least to take Ezetrol[*], or a lower dose of a statin with the

---

[*]Ezetrol/Zetia (ezetimibe) does not reduce the amount of cholesterol produced like statins. It does, however, prevent the

Ezetrol. When all attempts fail, he jots down a comment in my file – probably something to the effect 'patient refuses to take cholesterol lowering medication'. After all, if I do survive another heart attack, or worse yet, not survive another heart attack, he will have it documented that it was I who refused to take the his advice to lower my 'life threatening' cholesterol levels with statins. Bluntly stated, his butt will be covered. It was I who knowingly went against the cardiology world consensus.

He has been saving the lives of countless people over the last couple of decades. He was indoctrinated since his earliest days of medical school that cholesterol and fat are principal causes of heart disease. One would not expect that one Mike Stone would easily persuade a man of his stature that 'correlation when occurring is not causation' (regarding cholesterol and heart disease).

There is an important issue that the good professor never fails to bring up. It is also an issue that I have no rebuttal to offer him. The damage to my cardiovascular system resulting from 50 years of dietary abuse is a reality. The stent insertion did not cure my heart disease. It was simply a local solution to the most pressing problem to physically/mechanically open up a nearly completely

---

cholesterol from being absorbed from the small intestine into the bloodstream resulting in a decrease of cholesterol levels in the blood. Statins, despite well documented serious side effects at least do offer concrete cardio benefits. An article appearing in the New York Times March 31, 2008 entitled *Doubt Cast on 2 Drugs Used to Lower Cholesterol*, reported that ezetimibe 'failed to slow, and might have even sped up, the growth of fatty plaques in the arteries. Growth of those plaques is closely correlated with heart attacks and strokes.' Why am I not surprised??

blocked critical artery. The medications prescribed following my heart attack, including the statins, were not intended to cure the existing chronic medical condition. The sole intention of all of them was to help preserve the existing condition, and prevent further deterioration.

I also know as a non-medical person that this is the maximum that I can hope for even with all the changes I have made in my daily habits – the exercise, the dietary changes, reducing stress levels, etc. The elimination of trans-fats from my diet, being aware of omega-6 and omega-3 significance, less cooked foods, the freshly squeezed wheatgrass juice every morning, kefir, rejuvelac and all the other changes I discuss in this book will not *reverse* the 50 years of damage I caused to my cardiovascular system.

My existing cardiovascular system is not in an ideal condition to prevent an additional event from happening. The existing accumulated plaque is potentially susceptible to rupture – a common cause of blood clots. The stent also has its inherent potential risks. It is not something that I was born with; for all of its benefits it still remains a foreign metal object located in a very delicate area.

I mentioned in SASHA that I may one day consider undergoing EDTA Chelating therapy to clean up the blockages, and in a sense turn back the clock on the existing damage accumulated over my first 50 years. The question remains, is it truly effective? It is still considered to be controversial. And if chelating therapy, would it be the traditional intravenous procedure, or would the alternative oral chelating therapy be just as effective?[5]

Therefore, the question that begs to be answered is: to what extent exactly have I slowed down the further deterioration of my cardiovascular system by my lifestyle changes over the last number of years? I truly believe that had I changed my exercise/eating habits 30 years ago, my cardiovascular system would be in a vastly different state today. That, however, is not the relevant point today.

Despite vast improvements in my current health agenda, I do not totally abstain from modern conventional foods.   The   fact that I consume less of them, have eliminated the trans-fats from my diet as much as possible, and have added more raw/unrefined food only means that the rate of deterioration of my system has slowed down; I doubt that it has entirely stopped. Even if the rate has significantly decreased, over the years it is still slowly advancing.

What is it that really bothers me? I am not in denial. I do know that it is a possibility I may meet my cardiology professor not at one of our annual reunions, but rather when he on his feet and me on the bed again. The problem would not be him personally telling me 'See, I told you so'.

What bothers me is that for him this would be further proof of the lipid hypothesis. When on the statins my LDL cholesterol was 88, and according to all the other medical testing (statin induced mental and emotional dysfunction are not part of laboratory 'medical testing') I was in great shape. When taking myself off the statins, my cholesterol levels rose, which 'resulted' in another heart attack. Another statistic for the consensus -- additional proof that 'correlation is causation'.

It bothers me that even in this hypothetical situation, deep inside I know that I am right.

3

Uh-Oh – What's Wrong?

*Within 6 years after a recognized heart attack (MI), 18% of
men will have another heart attack, about 22%
will be disabled with heart failure, 8%
will have a stroke and 7% will
experience sudden death.*[6]

These are not especially encouraging statistics for us men. The statistics for women are even gloomier. Should I be especially happy that I am quickly approaching my sixth anniversary of my July 2001 heart attack?

December 2006:

Annual test results: I was surprised by the electrocardiogram (a.k.a. ECG or EKG) results during my stress test, which showed signs of 'not normal' during the final higher stress stages of the test.

What could have possibly caused these declines? I do realize I have been riding less; however, I have been walking more. Instead of driving to the parking lot at work, I park a 15-minute - half-hour walk away, depending whether I leave my house on time. The walk to work is, of course, not at an overly intensive pace, however, I do believe my recent past activity would still be classified as 'active'.

Could there be an effect because of the change to the normal daytime hours I had been working for most of my life? Although I no longer work the graveyard shift like I did for the first half of this year, I still don't get to bed before one a.m. most days of the week. Long gone are the days when I would be out at five a.m. I do miss that previous schedule, but this is the present reality.

I long ago abandoned the low-fat agenda; have I been over exaggerating my higher-fat diet?

My cardiology professor recommended that I do a thallium heart scan. So back to my health clinic to make the request to have the scan done at the appropriate hospital affiliated with my clinic.

A thallium heart scan is used to evaluate the blood supply to the heart muscle. A small amount of radioactive substance is injected into the bloodstream and a special camera is used to make an image of the blood flow to the heart. The radioactive substance is a radioisotope of the element thallium (thallium-201). This scan can identify areas of the heart that may have a poor blood supply as a result of damage from a previous heart attack or blocked coronary arteries.

January 2007

On the appointed day, I arrived at the hospital ready for my heart scan after a three-hour fast. As per instructions, I came happily equipped with a chocolate bar; it was that or come with some sour cream -- I didn't yet know the reason for this. The first order of business was the insertion an intravenous needle (IV line) into the vein on my right arm just below the elbow, the kind of IV that allows for injecting fluids multiple times. I then started what seemed to be a normal stress test on the treadmill.

Towards the latter stage of the test, which was already at a very rapid pace, a small amount of thallium-201 was injected into my IV line. Shortly after finishing the treadmill walk, I lay down under a special camera called a gamma scintillation camera. It made photographs from the gamma rays emitted by the thallium.

The purpose of the chocolate or sour cream: Radioisotope thallium-201 is a radioactive form of the element thallium (half-life of 73 hours). It was explained that it is advisable to ingest the fats in order to pad the liver from the radioactive material now circulating in the body.

The thallium attaches itself to red blood cells and is transported throughout the body in the bloodstream. It enters the heart muscle by way of the coronary arteries. The thallium can therefore reach only those areas of the heart with an adequate blood supply.

After this first set of gamma photographs taken shortly after my fast treadmill walk, I was instructed to return in another five hours. After returning, I was again injected with an additional shot of thallium. Within an hour, I was back under the scintillation camera for another round of gamma photographs, this time to get an image of the resting heart.

A normal thallium heart scan shows healthy blood flow through the coronary arteries without 'cold spots', both at rest and during exercise. A cold spot is an area where the heart tissue has been damaged (previous heart attack) or suffers from impaired circulation due to a blockage in the coronary arteries. It is an area the thallium has not reached, therefore does not show up on the gamma ray photograph. During exercise, the heart has to work harder and has a greater demand for blood. Cold spots that appear during exercise and not at rest usually indicate some blockage of the coronary arteries. People in this category are considered to be at a greater risk for future cardiac events such as heart attacks.

Results of the Heart Scan

The computerized printout of the December stress test did not come back positive; however, it did contain some comments regarding irregularities that are 'probably insignificant'. It was the sharp eye of my cardiology professor that determined that some of the squiggly lines on the EKG printout were not so insignificant as far as he was concerned. And indeed, the results of the thallium heart scan were positive. His recommendation: undergo an angiogram in the near future to verify the cause of the positive results of the heart scans.

Since discontinuing the statins three and a half years ago, I have been exercising regularly. I have discontinued ingesting partially hydrogenated foods (as much as possible) and therefore trans-fats. I have also discontinued the low-fat dairy agenda, with all of the artificial ingredients contained in them to keep them edible and 'dairy'. I have been eating more live foods, from naturally fermented raw milk products to wheatgrass juice. Have I been deceiving myself and causing additional blockages in my cardiovascular system?

To be continued…………..

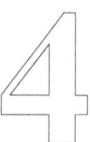

Raw Food & Enzymes

*The length of life is inversely proportional to the rate of
exhaustion of the enzyme potential of an organism*
Dr. Edward Howell[7]

In my generation the most important requirement
regarding healthy eating when growing up was to make
sure we were getting enough vitamins. Afraid of getting
a cold? 'Drink lots of orange juice because it has vitamin
C' we were told. I still remember a special kids' vitamin
that was taken as a small chocolate semi-sweet delicacy
every morning. That may even explain my long lasting
love affair with chocolate. I loved nearly every variation
of chocolate that there was - with the exception of any
chocolate containing raisins. I think my absolute favorite
was Three Musketeers. That did not prevent me from
consuming the competition whenever available: Hershey
Bars, Nestle's Crunch, even the coconut filled Peter Paul
Mounds bar and the like.

The next technical term while growing up regarding nutrition was minerals. What American kid did not start the day off with cereal for breakfast? It was definitely reassuring to read the message on the cereal box stating its contents were 'fortified' with vitamins and minerals.

I did not have any idea what the minerals were supposed to do, but having them supplied 'fortified' in my cereal definitely sounded reassuring. What kid could resist eating a 'fortified' cereal that had a picture of a baseball star printed on the front of the box? My favorite was mixing Wheaties and Cheerios together, letting them soak in the milk until mushy, and then eating it.

When growing up, how many times do you remember your mom telling you 'Eat your (whatever) to make sure you get enough enzymes'? Probably never. Enzymes? That sounds like a term for a chemist, or possibly a biologist. It was not for us laypeople, and definitely not a term that the average mom would be familiar with.

Why should I be concerned with enzymes? What you don't know can't hurt you, right? The problem is, by not knowing many things, I did have that heart attack at age 51, remember?

Merriam-Webster defines enzymes as 'any of numerous complex proteins that are produced by living cells and catalyze specific biochemical reactions at body temperatures'. In plain terms, 'catalyze specific biochemical reactions' translates to enzymes are the labor force of the body, catalyzing over 4,000 known biochemical reactions.[8] Enzymes are substances that make life possible. No mineral or vitamin can do any work without them. They are needed for **every** chemical reaction that takes place in our bodies.

Our bodies produce two types of enzymes:

Metabolic Enzymes

Metabolic enzymes run our bodies. A specific set of metabolic enzymes controls each organ in our bodies. These enzymes utilize the proteins, fats and carbohydrates that we eat to perform their functions.

Digestive Enzymes

Digestive enzymes have three main functions: to digest protein, carbohydrates and fat. Proteases are enzymes that digest protein, amylases digest carbohydrate, and lipases digest fat. Excessive production of digestive enzymes causes enlarged digestive organs, such as the pancreas.

There are hundreds of types of different known metabolic enzymes, and approximately two-dozen known digestive enzymes. Compared to vitamins and minerals, enzymes are the newest nutritional puzzle to be understood by nutritionists and scientists.

Many misconceptions apparently are still prevalent. Let's start with the basic Merriam-Webster definition: 'catalyze specific biochemical reactions'. A catalyst, by definition, is not consumed by the overall reaction. It accelerates or slows down the chemical reaction, nothing more.

It has been proven that the capacity of a living organism to make enzymes is limited and exhaustible. This negates the enzyme's status as a catalyst. It also follows that if the body is using its resources to produce digestive enzymes, it is at the expense of producing the metabolic enzymes. The best way to illustrate this would be to go back to my college days, and the famous Guns and Butter graph from Economics 101.

In a theoretical economy with the ability to produce two finite products and with a finite total production potential, a choice must be made between how much of each item to produce. In this example, as resources are used to produce more guns (military spending) the economy has less resources for the production of butter (domestic/food), and vice versa. The curve represents all possible choices the economy has at its disposal. The point here is that every choice has an opportunity cost; you can produce more of the first product only by giving up production of the second product. Assuming a given finite production potential, you cannot produce outside the curve.

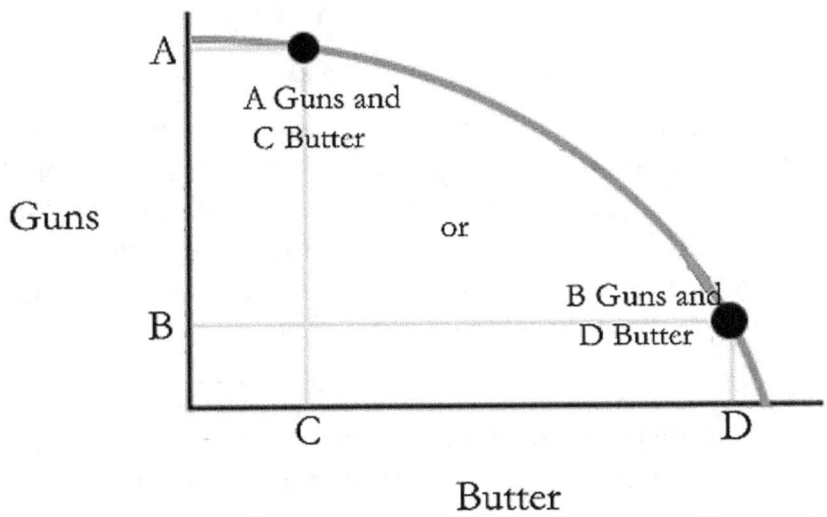

This model also demonstrates the production potential of body enzymes. When the body is forced to produce digestive enzymes at a particular time, it is at the expense of producing metabolic enzymes.

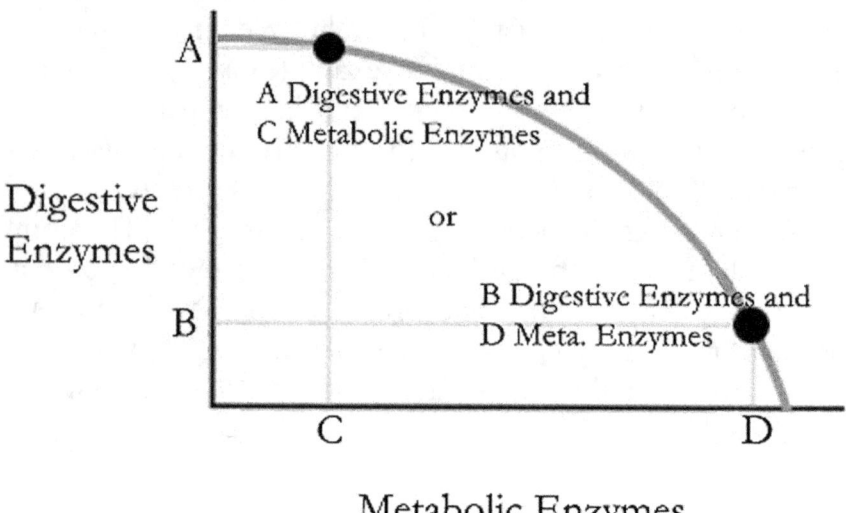

Metabolic Enzymes

Generally, digestion always has a high priority in the body's hierarchy of doing things. The production of the necessary digestive enzymes needed to digest the latest meal will have preference over the production of the hundreds of other metabolic enzymes necessary to run other important, if not critical, body processes.

Ultimately, man never comes out on top when tampering with nature. The case in point: tampering with the natural enzymes contained in raw food. Although our bodies are capable of producing digestive enzymes, it was not nature's intent that we do this function by ourselves. The enzymes contained in raw food play an important part in the pre-digestion of our food before it hits the stomach. This allows for a minimum production of supplementary digestive enzymes, and allows for maximum production of the important metabolic enzymes.

How are we destroying the enzymes in our food supply? Very bluntly, we cook it, and this is in addition to commercial food processing, which is often performed at high temperatures. Any prolonged wet-heat temperature over 118°F (47.8°C) kills 100% of the enzymes. This statement is so important that I will say it again. **Any prolonged wet-heat over 118°F (47.8°C) kills 100% of the enzymes!**

How hot is 118°F? An item at 117°F can be held in the hand with no problem. At 118° it is already too hot to handle. It starts to burn. This is significantly less than normal cooking temperatures; water boils at 212°F (100°C) and normal baking is at 300°F (149°C) - 400°F (204°C) dry heat. Enzymes can survive higher dry-heat temperatures -- but nothing even close to normal baking temperatures.

The Law of Adaptive Secretion of Digestive Enzymes

The Law of Adaptive Secretion of Digestive Enzymes governs characteristics of digestive enzyme production. This law states that an organism values its finite supply of enzymes and will make no more than are needed to do the job. Accordingly, the body produces the exact type and quantity of enzymes needed according to the protein, carbohydrate and fat makeup of the food eaten. Stated a bit more technically, the greater the amount of exogenous (outside) digestive enzymes we consume, the less production of the endogenous (internal) enzymes is required.

It naturally follows according to this law, ingesting natural enzymes already contained in the food we consume means the enzyme potential in our bodies can allot less activity to producing digestive enzymes and more to producing metabolic enzymes.

A good example to see how this works is to take an example directly from nature. Wild animals have no enzymes in their saliva. The bulk of the digestive enzymes needed to digest their prey are the enzyme banks existing in the prey itself. They need no enzymes in their saliva to start the predigesting process; these are ingested with each bite of the prey.

On a more domestic level, family dogs and cats that eat raw food exclusively also have no enzymes in their saliva. When fed cooked food, enzymes start showing up in their saliva within about a week; this is in full accordance with the law of adaptive secretion of digestive enzymes.

Uncooked foods contain an abundance of food enzymes, which correspond to the nutritional highlights of the food. For example, seeds, nuts dairy foods contain fat and higher concentration of lipase. Grains contain higher concentrations of amylase.

Is there a connection between the present state of my cardiovascular system and my own bodily enzyme activity? The two most potent enzymes secreted by the human body are amylase, which deals with the digestion of carbohydrates, and protease, which deals with the digestion of proteins. Our saliva contains a high concentration of amylase (how many times are we reminded to chew thoroughly?) while stomach juices contain protease.

Lipase, however, is present in weaker concentrations. As we grow older, enzyme activity grows weaker. Studies done over 50 years ago show a decrease in lipase levels and a definite alteration in the capacity of the aged human to handle fat.[9] Improvement in the fat utilization was exhibited by the subjects when later fed lipase. A later study demonstrated that there is a progressive decline of lipase in the blood of atherosclerosis patients with advancing middle and old age.[10] That certainly does not sound like good news for me. I am indeed considered to be an atherosclerosis patient and am now closer to 60 than to 50.

The easiest way to separate fat from its lipase enzyme is to destroy it by cooking. Without lipase to start the predigestion process, the fat remains unaltered for two to three hours in the stomach. All this occurs while the carbohydrates and proteins are being digested by the amylase and protease respectively. Again, lipase is not present in saliva, so no pre-digestion of fats can take place. As stated earlier, a greater necessity to produce digestive enzymes comes at the expense of the production of metabolic enzymes. This is definitely not great news for the 98 distinct known (metabolic) enzymes working in the arteries, each with a particular job to do.

This leads to the speculation that fat not pre-digested may not be properly metabolized (unhydrolyzed/partially digested) when it later reaches body tissues; the result is aggravated arterial linings and hardening of the arteries. This is basically what heart disease is all about!

In SASHA, I discussed how I discovered Dr. Dean Ornish and his best-selling book *Dr. Dean Ornish's Plan for Reversing Heart Disease*. Today, Ornish's low fat/high complex carbohydrate regimen is considered to be the arch rival of Dr. Robert Atkin's high fat/low carbohydrate diet plan. This book, however, as its name implies, is not specifically a diet plan; it is Ornish's comprehensive plan to reverse heart disease.

After learning about the vital importance of enzymes, I was curious what Dr. Ornish had to say about enzymes in general, and in particular, about lipase. I searched in the index for the word 'enzymes' and was surprised that it wasn't listed! Maybe he was more specific and indexed enzymes according to specific name. I looked for 'lipase' in the index, and again, no entry.

Suddenly I understood the 'genius' of Ornish's plan to combat heart disease. Cardiovascular disease is the epidemic of the modern Western world. The ingesting of copious amounts of commercially processed fats devoid of enzymes in the Western diet is indeed a source of heart disease.

Dr. Ornish found an innovative solution to 'solve' this problem. For most people in today's modern world, obtaining and consuming necessary healthy fat in the form nature intended with enzymes intact is not feasible. His solution to circumvent the real problem: simply eliminate almost all the fats!

The emphasis in today's cardio world is not on prevention; it is on repair. And why not? Modern technologies can do wonders with our precious bodies with prescription medications and operations. Angiogram, angioplasty, stents and bypass operations are great tools to fix anyone who has managed to clog up his/her arteries, assuming of course that they make it to the hospital on time. What is sad is that this is considered 'normal' in our modern civilization.

Take someone with a Rolls Royce that gasses it up with kerosene instead of the proper octane gasoline. If it later does not run as it should, but he has a great mechanic who can fix it, would this seem normal? No? Why then is his Rolls more precious than our own precious bodies?

Would it not make more sense to consume foods with more live enzymes, or even supplement meals with enzymes rather than try and control the damage with medications or fix the problem later using intrusive medical procedures?

Are we like Pottenger's cats?

From 1932 to 1942, Dr. Francis Marion Pottenger, Jr. conducted a controlled experiment[11] on generations of cats (total 900 cats) to determine the effects of heat-processed food them. The cats were divided into groups. All the groups were supplied the same basic minimal diet (meat, milk and cod liver oil), but the major portions of the diets were varied. One group ate raw meat and raw milk exclusively, a natural food for cats. The other groups were fed processed milk: pasteurized, evaporated and condensed milk, with either raw or cooked meat.

All generations of the raw meat/milk groups remained healthy throughout their normal life spans. The first generation of all the other processed-food groups developed degenerative diseases and illnesses towards the end of their lives. The next generation of these groups developed degenerative diseases and illnesses in the middle of their lives and started losing their coordination. The third generation of the processed food groups developed degenerative diseases in the beginning of their lives and many died before six months of age. Bones became soft and the cats suffered from adverse personality changes.

Males became docile, less interested in mating while females became more aggressive.

There was no fourth generation in any of the processed food groups. Either the third generation parents were sterile or the fourth generation cats died before birth. Again, this is in direct contrast to the fourth generation of the cats on the raw food/milk diet, which remained healthy throughout their normal lifespan.

Dr. Pottenger concluded that a diet consisting exclusively of raw milk and raw meat was the only adequate food that insured optimal health for the cats. Cats on the all-raw diet showed good bone structure with excellent bone density. They had wide palates with plenty of room for properly aligned teeth. They exhibited a shiny coat and were free of disease. In addition, these cats reproduced with ease and were gentle and easy to handle. The cats eating processed foods (meat/milk) developed physical degeneration that escalated with each successive generation.

Of special interest to those of you who do purchase and consume raw milk, Dr. Pottenger also showed that not all-raw milk is created equally.

> *In comparing the experimental effects on cats of a diet including raw milk from fresh feed cows and those of a diet including raw milk from dry feed cows, we find that the cats fed raw milk from dry feed cows show similar deficiencies as those fed pasteurized milk.*[12]

People are people, cats are cats, but…

Why should I be influenced by a study that was done on cats over 70 years ago? As in the computer era, 70 years is also a long time as far as medical advancement is concerned. In addition, how many people do you know that have received a kitten from a domesticated cat eating processed food and watched the kitten grow older and give birth to litter after litter of apparently healthy kittens? You probably know many people that fit this description; and those cats are all brought up on commercially processed food.

That said how is the research of Dr. Pottenger applicable to us today? I certainly have not noticed an abundance of domesticated malformed dying cats roaming around my own neighborhood. How were Pottenger's cats similar to us? How did they differ?

We are both warm-blooded. We are both mammals. We reproduce in a similar fashion, give birth after a fixed pregnancy period, and nurse the newborns.

On the other hand, we humans by nature are omnivores (capable of eating meat protein and vegetation). Cats are carnivores (meat eaters). This alone dictates that dietary requirements of humans will not be the same as cats.

> *This evolutionary development has resulted in more stringent nutritional requirements for cats than for omnivores such as the rat, dog, and man.*[13]

The different dietary requirements are of course dictated by the differences in our biological systems. As an example, for us humans, taurine is a nonessential amino acid, meaning that it is manufactured from other amino acids in the liver. It does not have to be obtained directly through the diet. On the other hand, taurine, found only in animal products, is an important *essential* amino acid for the cat.[14]

Some of the abnormalities displayed by Pottenger's cats can possibly be attributed to taurine deficiency, such as poor reproductive performance and neurological abnormalities. This could possibly be explained by the cooking of the meat, which destroyed the taurine in the food fed to the cats.[15]

Dr. Pottenger studied cats. As stated previously, the cats eating raw food/milk were healthy and properly developed generation after generation.

Dr. Weston A. Price studied people throughout the whole world. The 'primitive' societies eating traditional foods were free of chronic disease and dental decay; they were strong and produced healthy children generation after generation. Dr. Price observed that modern civilization eating refined grains, canned foods, pasteurized milk and sugars suffered from degenerative illnesses, infertility, crooked teeth, narrowed faces, deformities of bone structure and susceptibility to every sort of medical problem.[16]

This same degeneration observed by Dr. Price in tribes and villages that had abandoned traditional foods was also observed by Dr. Pottenger for the cats eating heat-processed (cooked/pasteurized) food.

No, people are not cats; however Dr. Pottenger summed this up quite nicely:

> *While no attempt will be made to correlate the changes in the animals studied with malformations found in humans, **the similarity is so obvious that parallel pictures will suggest themselves.***[17] (Bold emphasis is mine.)

What do **you** think?

How do we then conserve our finite potential of enzymes? Besides killing enzymes found in natural food by cooking, our own enzymes are used up faster during certain illnesses, during extremely hot or cold weather, and during strenuous exercise. We have all heard of Eskimos. Eskimos have been notorious for enjoying excellent health by eating a raw diet. The name 'Eskimo' itself is based on an American Indian language meaning 'he eats it raw' or 'eaters of raw meat', depending on which dialect is used. In the case of Eskimos, raw food means raw meat – their cholesterol levels are sky high, but heart disease if virtually non-existent.

A Western culture family that adapted eating raw food as the standard in the house, and not as the exception, is the Boutenko[18] family -- today known as the Raw Family. In the mid-nineties, different members of the Boutenko family suffered from a variety of illnesses, such as obesity, depression, rheumatoid arthritis, severe hyperthyroid, juvenile diabetes and asthma. After going on a totally raw diet, all those health problems were miraculously healed. We will return to the (Victoria) Boutenko family in chapter 11.

Is going on a 100% raw diet practical for most people? The answer is 'no' despite the enzyme conservation and other health benefits of doing so. Raw food is digested in less than half the time as cooked food. The extended hours of digestion creates rotting and intestinal illnesses.

What percentage of raw food in our diet should we strive for? 90%? 70%? How much? The natural health care nutritionist Hanna Kroeger[19] mentions figures of 50%

raw and 50% cooked for fighting diseases. She also claims that enzyme supplements are just as valid as adding vitamins and minerals to our diets.

Do I even approach 100% raw food? Not even close. Although I do strive to increase this percentage, I cannot really say if I am at 30%, 40%, 50%, or 60%. It is the purpose of this book to show how small adjustments in our eating habits can make a big difference in improving these percentages.

5

Why is Raw Food so Unappealing?

I want my food dead. Not sick, not dying, dead.
Oscar Wilde

Why is it that so many people find the idea of eating raw food repelling? It all boils down to preconceptions of what we think food should look and smell like. As it turns out, these preconceptions are not at all objective; in fact they are very subjective.

There are many clichés out there – 'you can't judge a book by its cover', or 'beauty is in the eye of the beholder'. We even have a rhyming expression in Hebrew that says 'Ol Taam v-ol rai-och, ain ma lhitvaka-och' which translates literally to 'regarding taste and smell, there is nothing to argue about'. Stated more abruptly: one person's sense of what is aesthetic, smells nice or is tasty, may be utterly disgusting to someone else.

To prove my point, I have two actual examples involving real people. I won't mention the names and relationship to 'protect the innocent'. The first example

29

involves something I consider to be a real delicacy, tongue. There are several different ways one can eat tongue.

One option: cut very, very thin, stacked nice and thick between two slices of fresh rye bread smeared with mustard -- literally heaven on Earth. One of my favorite places to eat a tongue sandwich when visiting New York was always the Second Avenue Kosher Delicatessen. The Second Ave Deli, as it was commonly known, had a long and interesting history. Abe Lebewohl, an Ukrainian immigrant who arrived in the United States in 1950, worked there as a waiter in what was then a 12-seat capacity coffee shop for several years.

In 1954, Mr. Lebewohl and several partners at the time purchased the delicatessen. As fate would have it, Mr. Lebewohl was murdered in 1996, a daylight robbery in which he was depositing the previous day's receipts. The restaurant doors were unfortunately closed for good in 2006 by its then owner, Jack Lebewohl, the younger brother of Abe. The closure was the result of a rent increase dispute with the building's new landlord.

I will state that there is a yearly ritual when we do eat tongue; it saves me the necessity of traveling all the way to New York just to have a tongue sandwich! Anyone who has ever participated in a Jewish Passover Seder[*] knows that before you get to the main meal, there is a long ceremony beforehand where various symbolic foods are blessed. In fact there is a special Passover plate that is divided in sections to hold the different symbolic items.

---

[*] The Passover Seder is a Jewish ritual feast which takes place on the first evening of Passover holiday in Israel, and on the first and second evenings of Passover in the Jewish Diaspora. The feast includes reading the Haggadah, which contains the complete Seder service.

Here in Israel, it is the tradition in families of Sephardic origin** (Esty's family immigrated to Israel from Iraq in the early 1950's) to also have a ceremony preceding the festive Rosh Hashanah (New Year) meal. It is much shorter than the Passover ceremony; however, it does have various symbolic foods on which blessings are said. One of these blessings is:

yehi ratzon m'lifanecha adonoi elokanu v'elovei avoteinu sh-nehiye l'rosh v'lo l'znav.....

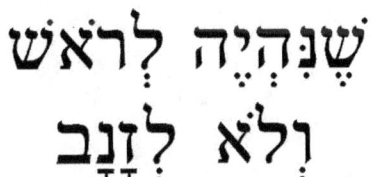

שֶׁנִּהְיֶה לְרֹאשׁ
וְלֹא לְזָנָב

which basically translates to 'G-d willing we should all be like the head, and not the tail'. Following the blessing, we then eat something representing the 'head'. In our family it is a portion of boiled tongue, sliced into inch wide sections, a true delicacy.

What is all this leading to? This may seem like a benign point; however much of the food we consume on the plates in front of us doesn't always resemble what its raw material looks like before processing and packaging.

The case in point – real people, no names...we will refer to them as couple A and couple B. Couple A invited couple B over to dinner. Mrs. A was still in the kitchen

---

**By strict definition a Sephardi is a Jew whose forefathers originated from Portugal or Spain. In a broader sense, the term has come to also include Jews of Arabic and Persian backgrounds. In present day usage it has become an umbrella term for any Jewish person who is not Ashkenazi (Ashkenazis are descendants of Jews from Germany, Poland, Austria and Eastern Europe).

when couple B arrived a bit early. Mrs. A still had a large tongue cooking in the pot.

It may seem redundant to state that tongue is called 'tongue' because it originates in a cow's mouth! When couple B saw the complete cow's tongue still in the pot and as yet uncut into individual portions, the sight of it sickened them. It simply ruined their appetite for the entire evening. What is interesting is this same couple B that could not stomach seeing a cooked cow's tongue in the pot loves eating lobsters.

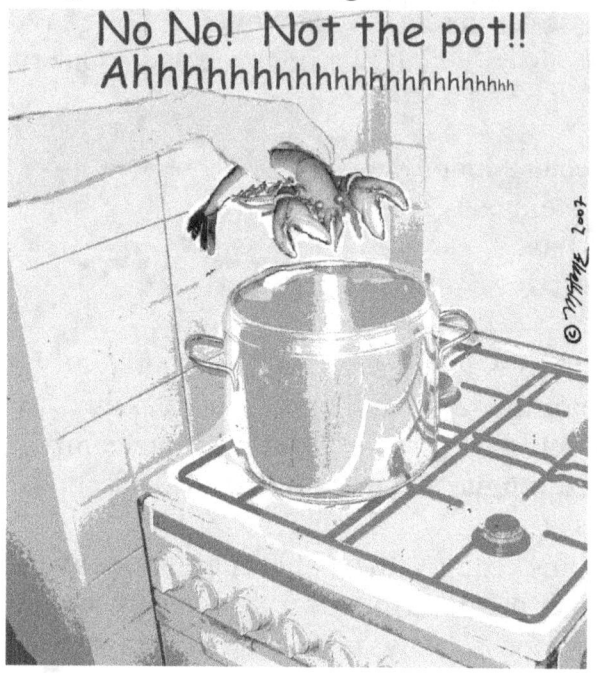

For those of you who may not be totally familiar with lobsters, they are undoubtedly one of the ugliest creatures on the planet. When I was younger, they would remind me of what a giant spider might look like, with armor and pinchers. The whole procedure of eating a lobster starts with its purchase, while it is alive and well, swimming in a glass-lined pool waiting to be bought. The buyer looks them all over, even looks the lobster straight in the eye, and decides, 'I want you'. Lobsters are tossed into a boiling red-hot pot for steaming, meaning that the first lobster to hit the pot has a good chance of hitting some boiling water before getting steamed live.

This procedure is accompanied with jokes to the tune of 'woo - listen to the lobster yelling'. I wonder if other lobsters do actually hear their comrades screaming from the pot. And of course, the culmination of this whole process -- the actual eating of the lobster.

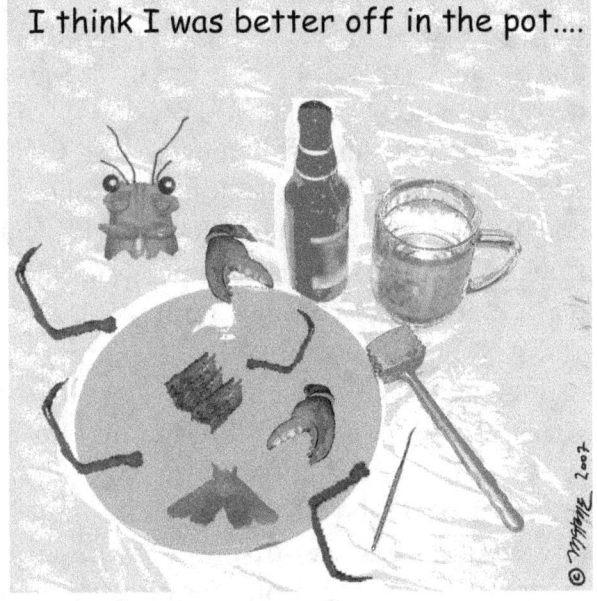

I think I was better off in the pot....

For someone who has never seen this ritual, it is grotesque. The process starts with literally ripping off its pinchers and its legs. To carve out the meat inside the armor you have something that resembles a nut clipper, and if you have trouble getting into the claw, you have a wooden hammer to crack the armored shell. Then of course there is opening up the lobster from its belly side, and scooping out the lobster meat from all of its dismembered parts. I did previously mention grotesque, didn't I? What's the point? To couple B, seeing a very natural complete cow's tongue cooking in a large pot was unbearable.

The whole process of purchasing, cooking live and then dismembering the lobster to them is an accepted way of preparing and eating food.

The second example is similar. Person C (yes, another name change) came over to Israel for a visit from the States. One evening Esty prepared a nice fish dinner. Again here we see the differences between different cultures, and how each views the same situation in different ways. It is very acceptable in Israel, in restaurants and in the home as well, to serve fish complete and intact. This is not to say that you cannot obtain a fish fillet that has been de-boned and sliced up into portions.

A complete fish means just that. It comes served with its head and eyes intact. When person C saw the cooked fish on the plate 'looking back at her', she simply freaked out. And what's special about this example? This particular person enjoys going out and ordering steamed crabs. The procedure for steaming, dismembering and eating crabs is similar to that described for lobsters -- and why not, they are in the same family known as crustaceans.

The standard procedure is going to a crab house with family or a bunch of friends. The table is lined with either newspapers, or a disposable paper tablecloth. What distinguishes a crab house from a steak house, for example, is that at a crab house everyone puts on bib.

No, I do not mean a napkin on the lap type of protection, but a bib that you tie around your neck to keep your shirt clean. Why the bib? When your neighbor on either side starts clobbering dismembered crab parts with the wooden hammer to break the outer armor shell, pieces of meat, shell and any other internal parts can start flying around the table.

Again, this to some people is a normal, pleasant, acceptable way of eating a meal, while seeing a complete uncut fish with its head still on is considered to be unbearable. And so it is with many people's preconceptions of eating anything raw for the first time 'Yuck! I can't eat that! It's not cooked!'

I admit that the first time I cut into a steak that was totally raw, I also had a similar feeling.* However, after the first small bite, chewing it up, and swallowing that first piece, the apprehension quickly disappeared. What we conceive to be aesthetic food and what isn't is all in the mind.

This concludes Introduction to Eating Raw Food 101.....

---

* Although cooking kills much of the healthy attributes of food, it also eliminates many harmful aspects, bacteria etc. Raw food must be 'prepared correctly' and obtained from reputable sources.

Pasteur – Hero or Villain?

*The general public, however intelligent, are struck only by
that which it takes little trouble to understand*
Antoine Béchamp[20]

Part 1: Louis Pasteur, Pasteurization – Brief Review

Louis Pasteur, the famous French microbiogist and
chemist, was born in 1822. He is best known for
developing a system of heat application to control
fermentation, which resulted in the non-spoilage of wine
and beer. His heat application involved raising the
temperature of wine to kill the specific living
microorganisms that cause spoilage. This process, which
ultimately immortalized his name universally and is today
commonly associated with milk, is known as
'pasteurization'.

His other major claim to fame was his germ theory
of disease, technically known as the pathogenic theory of
medicine. The theory proposes that microorganisms are the

cause of many diseases. Although highly controversial when first proposed, it is now a cornerstone of modern medicine and clinical microbiology, leading to widespread usage of prescription medicines and antibiotics. He also created the first vaccine for rabies.

His academic resume was impressive:

1848: Professor of Physics at Dijon Lycee
1849: Professor of Chemistry at Strasbourg University
1854: Dean of the College of Science in Lille.
1856: Administrator and director of scientific studies of the École Normale Supérieure.
1862: Member of French Academy of Science

Pasteur won the Leeuwenhoek medal, microbiology's highest honor, in 1895, the year of his death.

The remains of Pasteur are interred at the chapel of the Pasteur Institute, Marnes-la-Coquette, France. One of the walls of the chapel summarizes the accomplishments attributed to him.

1857: Fermentations
1862: So-called 'Spontaneous Generation'
1863: Studies in Wine
1865: Disease of Silkworms
1871: Studies in Beer
1877: Virulent Microbic Diseases
1880: Vaccinating Viruses
1885: Prophylaxis of Rabies

Interestingly, his list of accomplishments at the chapel does not include any specific reference to milk.

Pasteurization

Pasteurization is the process of heating food in order to kill harmful organisms such as bacteria, viruses, protozoa, molds, and yeasts. Pasteurization, unlike sterilization, is not intended to kill all microorganisms in the food; it aims to achieve a five-log reduction (0.00001 times the original) in the number of viable organisms, reducing their number so they are unlikely to cause disease.

This assumes of course that the pasteurized product is refrigerated and consumed before its expiration date. Today, pasteurization is typically associated with milk/milk products. The justification for pasteurizing milk was that it often became contaminated while being handled on its way to the consumer.

Pasteur became famous for saving the French wine industry when 'pasteurizing' wine to keep it from spoiling. The feat was immortalized on the chapel wall – 1863. Again, the wall contains no reference to milk! Interestingly, when was the last time you bought a bottle of wine labeled as 'pasteurized'?

Pasteurization methods for milk are usually standardized and controlled by national food safety agencies, such as the USDA in the United States and the Food Standards Agency in the United Kingdom.

Today, there are two widely used methods of pasteurizing milk:

HTST - High Temperature/Short Time

HTST is by far the most common method. Milk labeled simply as pasteurized is usually treated with the HTST method. HTST involves holding the milk at a temperature of 145°F (62°C) for half an hour or 161.5°F (72°C) for at least 15 seconds. The HTST pasteurization processes must be designed so that the milk is heated evenly, and no part of the milk is subject to a shorter time or a lower temperature. HTST pasteurized milk typically has a refrigerated shelf life of two to three weeks.

UHT - Ultra-High Temperature

UHT involves holding the milk at a temperature of 280-285°F (138-141°C) for at least two seconds. This process actually sterilizes the milk. UHT pasteurized milk can last in the refrigerator for two to three months. When UHT pasteurization is combined with sterile handling and container technology, the milk can even be stored unrefrigerated for long periods. For those of you who like to drink UHT milk, Dr. Paul Kouchakoff determined in 1930 that the critical temperature above which milk becomes recognized by the white cells of the blood as an enemy of the body is only 88.3°C (191°F).[21]

There are different pasteurization standards for different dairy products, depending on the fat content and the intended usage. For example, the pasteurization standards for fluid milk differ from the standards for cream; the standards (heat used) for pasteurizing cheese are designed to preserve the phosphatase enzyme, which aids in curing the cheese.

Part 2: Pasteur and Pfizer – are there similarities?

"Louis Pasteur, one of the legendary figures in the history of science, lied about his research, stole ideas from a competitor and was deceitful in ways that would now be regarded as scientific misconduct if not fraud."[22] This is part of a book review that appeared in the New York Times reviewing *The Private Science of Louis Pasteur*, by Dr. Gerald L. Geison of Princeton University. Big deal! For 100 years since Pasteur's death until the publication of the New York Times article, Pasteur was a world hero, the scientist's scientist. So what if he cut some corners here and there. Why should that bother me? Don't things like happen in other professions? For instance, let's look at some recent journalism scandals.

Who doesn't remember *Jimmy's World* a phony story about a child heroin addict? The story appeared in the Washington Post on September 29, 1980 and won a Pulitzer Prize for reporter Janet Cooke. The prize was later returned.

Newspaper reporter Jayson Blair resigned from the New York Times after admitting he faked and plagiarized dozens of stories. Jack Kelley, the ex-USA Today reporter resigned following allegations that he faked major stories.[23] I do not feel that Jack Kelley dramatically changed my life, or Jason Blair, or even Janet Cooke, who initially walked away with the Pulitzer. All of their events occurred within the last 30 years. Louis Pasteur died over 100 years ago. I should not have to be concerned if he plagiarized or lied about his research. Or should I be?

Louis Pasteur, while still alive, never released his laboratory notes. He left them to his family with instructions never to release them. With the death of his last male descendant, a grandson in 1975, they became the property of the French National Library.

Professor Geison was the first person to thoroughly review those notes; he spent 15 years studying more than 10,000 pages of lecture notes and lab workbooks.

It was not Geison's intent to discredit Pasteur or his contributions to science, but he did want to present the unadorned truth. The American Association for the History of Medicine awarded its 1996 William H. Welch Medal to Professor Geison for his suburb investigative work.

The question remains if humanity had to wait the 80 or so years following Pasteur's death to fully understand how he conducted and publicized his research. Does it significantly affect our lives today?

With today's modern technology, anyone, and I do mean anyone, can write and publish a book. You can find books on virtually every subject imaginable, with all views possible represented. Take for example the underlying subject matter of this book. There are almost an infinite number of books claiming to explain the 'real cause' of heart disease. There are a myriad of books siding with the current consensus that cholesterol is the main culprit in causing heart disease, and a growing number claiming exactly the opposite.

Anyone can write a book? I am a classic example. I am not connected to the medical profession, and here I am writing not my first book, but my second book regarding a very serious and relevant health issue. SASHA being a self-published paperback does not meet the requirements to appear on the New York Times bestseller list, nevertheless, it has obtained ranking on the major international sales outlets: Amazon, Amazon England, Amazon Germany, Barnes & Nobles, etc.

Yes, the electronic age has made it very easy for anyone not only to market a book, but for the actual writing as well. I remember when the first personal computers hit the market. The big key on the right-hand side of the keyboard was not marked with a '◄⌐' as today, but with the letters 'CR'. Ask any 15-year-old computer whiz today what the CR stands for. I doubt that very few, if any, will give the correct answer. It stands for 'Carriage Return'.

For those of my generation, the CR will bring back the memory of those old Smith-Corona heavy typewriters, pounding away at those mechanical heavy keys, where each hit of the key moved the carriage physically one letter width to the right. You would arrive to the end of the line; a small bell would ring signaling for the typist to finish the present word being typed and then Trockkkk! The right-hand leaves the keyboard to slam the carriage return lever back to the left-hand side of the typewriter. The Trockkk would also advance the page to the next line according to the line spacing previously set mechanically, and the new line begins.

OOOOOPS -- you made a mistake -- advance the paper forward, use your eraser shield to expose the misprinted letter and protect adjacent letters, erase it, move the paper back into the exact location on the page, and then retype the new letter.

Typewriters also advanced with technology. I remember when we had an IBM Selectric electric typewriter. Instead of having to hen peck the heavy keys, the electric touch made the actual act of typing similar to the light touch-typing of the modern computer keyboard. On the IBM Selectric, the paper remained static. There was a small metal ball embedded with all the letters, numbers and symbols that ran back and forth in place of the carriage and typed the letter. Even correcting errors became easier. Quick drying white correction fluid and the dry 'correct-o-type' sheets replaced the eraser shields and erasers.

Today, in the computer age, typing and basic editing have become a no-brainer. OOOOPS, you made a mistake? No problem. Use your mouse to go directly to the error and retype. Change around the order? No problem. Simply 'cut and paste' and rearrange to your heart's content. Turn on the spell checker, and automatically some misprints and mistakes are clearly identified.

Writing and publishing a book was not always as easy as it is today. There was a time when a writer had to be extremely dedicated in order to present a finished manuscript in acceptable format. As a prerequisite, the subject matter of the book had to be worthy of the effort in order to find a reputable publisher.

No, humankind did not have to wait until the computer age and the Internet to read a book regarding Pasteur's method of science back in the 1800's. One of the first books published that took a serious look at the work of Pasteur in an unfavorable light was *Béchamp or Pasteur* by Ethel Douglas. The book was first published in 1923 and later revised and published in 1932 – that is more than half a century before Pasteur's lab notes were made public! Ms. Douglas had much to say regarding all of Pasteur's accomplishments listed on the wall of the chapel of the Pasteur Institute at Marnes-la-Coquette. For instance:

We have already seen, firstly, that in regard to fermentation in general and vinous fermentation in particular, as also in regard to silkworm disease, it is impossible to deny that Pasteur plagiarized Béchamp. Secondly, we have seen that Pasteur's experiments were insufficient to defeat the theory of spontaneous generation and that they never satisfied Sponteparists, such as Pouchet, LeBon and Batian.[24]

It is not my intention to go into any additional technical detail regarding her revelations; what bothers me is the monster that Pasteur ultimately created.

Pasteurism has become a vested interest, and one, unfortunately, supported by that powerful trade union – the Medical Fraternity[25]

Dr. Guylaine Lanctôt wrote a book called *The Medical Mafia*. The title is self-explanatory; she delves into numerous existing medical issues. Regarding her comments about Pasteur:

Pasteur was ambitious, an opportunist? He was also a genius in the art of promoting himself, and he plagiarized, and then vulgarized, the work of Béchamp. He stole the idea of small organisms being responsible, but he only revealed a small part of Béchamp's discoveries. Pasteur proclaimed that these small organisms only came from the outside. He forgot to mention that, once exposed to air, germs and other morbid (abnormal) microzymes lose their virulence very rapidly. **And this deceit has been perpetuated ever since.**[26] (Bold emphasis is mine.)

The point I am leading up to can best be described by Shelley and Denie Hiestand in *Electrical Nutrition: A revolutionary approach to eating that awakens the body*:

> *Béchamp, a man without public savvy, argued all his life that disease was caused by disharmony and imbalance of the body's natural microflora; but his boss,* **Pasteur, who was being funded by his friends in the rapidly growing pharmaceutical industry**, *promoted the idea that bacteria caused disease and that bacteria could be killed by drugs.* **Our entire germ-based microorganism-killing pharmaceutical industry grew from this erroneous scientific premise.**
>
> *On his deathbed, Pasteur apologized for deliberately taking Béchamp's research out of context so that* **his institute could benefit from the funding that was coming from the newly emerging drug companies.** *In fact, he admitted that he was wrong and that Béchamp was right. By then, however,* **the drug companies and their 'kill-the-germs-at-all-cost' system is a direct legacy of this lie.**[27] (Bold emphasis is mine.)

What is the connection between Pasteur and Pfizer? Pfizer is the world's largest drug maker. Its 2006 revenues totaled over $48.3 billion.[28] Its research and development spending for the same year reached almost $7.6 Billion.[29] It manufactures Lipitor, the world's top-selling medicine, with almost $12.9 billion in annual sales.[30]

Lipitor (atorvastatin) is a member of the statin family of medicines. Statin sales in the world depend upon prolonging the 'validity' of the (blood) lipid hypothesis. Just as Pasteur benefited greatly from marketing erroneous scientific results, so has Pfizer been benefiting from the existing world belief that high cholesterol causes heart disease (lipid hypothesis).

Why did I particularly pick on Pfizer? No particular reason, simply because they are the largest and most well-known pharmaceutical company on the planet. Dr. Duane Graveline,[31] a flight surgeon and former astronaut, was a pioneer in publicizing the serious side effects caused by Lipitor which caused his two bouts of transient global amnesia (TGA).

I could have just as easily picked Merck, the manufacturer of Zocor (simvastatin) and Mevacor (lovastatin). I could have picked Bayer, the manufacturer of Baycol (cerivastatin), which was withdrawn from the market in 8/2001 due to too many fatalities; or Novartis, the manufacturer of Lescol (fluvastatin). I could have picked AstraZeneca, the manufacturer of Crestor (rosuvastatin).

I could have even picked my 'favorite', Bristol-Myers Squibb, the manufacturer of Pravachol (Pravastatin). It was a locally marketed version of Pravastatin known as Lipidal that so disrupted my professional and personal life and inspired the writing of SASHA.

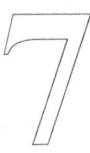

Post Pasteur

*There are two kinds of statistics, the kind you look up,
and the kind you make up.*
Rex Stout

During my university days, I took several statistics courses, which included of course lessons regarding statistical testing. I remember the time when flash bulbs were still used when taking indoor pictures. The flash bulb was basically a very small light bulb; it could only be used once. The one time flash occurrence when taking the picture was the bulb's entire purpose of existence. One picture and that was it; then to the trash can and flash bulb heaven. As we learned in statistical testing, testing all the bulbs would certainly be counterproductive, as all the bulbs would be destroyed in the test.

Calcium

The successful test of pasteurization for milk is to verify that all of the enzyme phosphatase in the milk has been totally destroyed.[32] The one small problem with this test is that phosphatase is essential for the proper absorption of calcium. Do you wonder why you encounter more and more people that suffer from osteoporosis? Proper calcium levels in the body are essential for strong bones and teeth, regulating muscle and heart function among other functions. Sure, calcium is abundant in other food products besides dairy products. However, if they are also cooked, then the natural occurring phosphatase is still destroyed. Incidentally, eating foods 'fortified' with calcium doesn't guarantee that your body will automatically be able to absorb and process this form of calcium effectively. Synthetic nutrients can be toxic.[33]

Vitamins

It was stated as early as 1942 that the cows of the country produce as much vitamin C as does the entire national citrus crop, but most of it is lost as a result of pasteurization.[34] The vitamin C that does survive the pasteurization process is diluted even more in many supermarkets even before it reaches your refrigerator. Most milk is packaged in translucent plastic jugs. Many supermarkets market milk in refrigerated sections lighted by fluorescent lighting. Fluorescent lighting has been shown to destroy half of the vitamin C content of the milk.[35] Pasteurization has also been shown to destroy vitamin A (necessary to assimilate protein[36]) and greatly reduces the amount of vitamin B complex.[37]

Digestion of Fats

Pasteurization destroys lipase,[38] the enzyme that aids in the digestion of fats. Triglycerides are the main constituents of milk fat.[39] How often are we told after blood testing that our 'trigs are too high'? Carbohydrates and proteins start undergoing the pre-digestion process in the upper stomach thanks to salivary amylase and pepsin. While this is occurring, the fats, devoid of lipase, remain unaltered in the stomach for up to several hours after swallowing. When hitting the hydrochloric acid in the stomach without the benefit of pre-digestion, the fats may be improperly metabolized when they ultimately reach body tissues.[40]

Milk Sugar

Lactase is an enzyme that breaks down the milk sugar lactose into galactose and glucose.[41] Pasteurization inactivates the naturally occurring lactase in raw milk. It also destroys galactase, the enzyme needed to break down galactose. How often do we hear of people being 'lactose intolerant'?

Selenium

Selenium is an antioxidant mineral that helps regulate nitric oxide in the arteries, which is of prime importance in preventing heart disease.[42] Pasteurization reduces the availability of selenium in commercial cow's milk by 10%.[43]

Dirty, Dead Milk

Pasteurization is an excuse for the sale of low-quality, dirty milk. It discourages the effort to produce clean milk.[44] It all starts with the personal hygiene of the cow herself. As Dr. William Douglas II aptly stated, "A cow is not a cat...Cows are not neat. Their personal hygiene would embarrass a pig."[45] Producing clean milk would entail making the effort to physically clean up the teats of the cow properly before each milking. This takes time and money.

Truthfully, it is hard to blame the modern commercial dairy in this day and age. In order to survive, it has to maximize production and minimize costs. The nutritional quality of his final product is of little, if any, concern. And why should it be? The dairyman's milk totally loses its personal identity once it leaves his diary and mixes with the milk of possibly hundreds of other diaries at the processing plant, some diaries likely much filthier than his own.

The pasteurization process involves raising the temperature of the milk to high temperatures not necessarily only once, but possibly several times to kill off all the harmful 'ingredients'. Some processes even involve steam cleaning.[46] Stated differently, due to the pasteurization process, most of the harmful junk in the milk that we would not want to drink is also dead by the time it hits our refrigerators. This is sort of like a built-in booby prize.

Pasteurized milk is therefore essentially dead milk. Pasteurization kills the natural enzymes present in raw milk and alters the protein[47] and fat. Raw milk sours when not refrigerated. Pasteurized milk, with all of its enzymes killed and protein and fat altered by the heating process, simply rots. It putrefies; it is dead before it reaches your refrigerator.

The Ultimate 'Cat' Scan

Who am I to state that raw milk is alive, and pasteurized milk is essentially dead? After all, what do I know? I am only human. In order to test this out, we will go to a non-human, however, a connoisseur of milk and milk products. This will be a true 'cat' scan, supervised by Nivi and Gray, two of the family's cats.

Nivi is intelligent as far as cats go. When hungry, instead of just meowing she jumps up to the kitchen window, stands on her hind legs and scratches continuously on the window while looking me straight in the eye. You can see Nivi in action at the bottom of web page http://www.heartrecovey.net/books2.html. Gray is Nivi's grandson (as far as I remember – it's easy to lose track…).

This 'cat' scan is opposed to the more familiar CAT (Computed Axial Tomography) scan where digital geometry processing is used to generate a three-dimensional image of internal organs.

For this particular cat scan, I prepared two glasses of milk. One glass was raw (unpasteurized) goat's milk; the other was a glass of standard HTST 3% carton milk purchased at the supermarket.

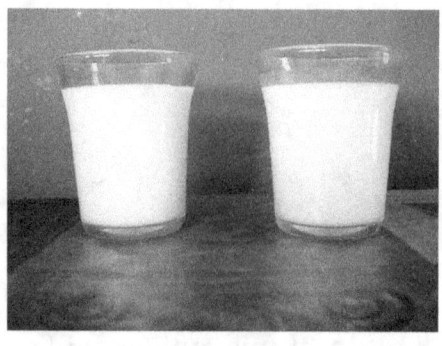 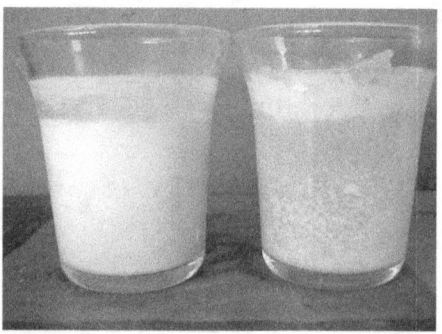

Day 1: On the left is standard 3% fresh pasteurized homogenized (cow) milk. On the right, fresh raw (unpasteurized) goat's milk. They look identical.

A week later at room temperature, the pasteurized milk has started to evaporate. The fresh goat's milk has separated into whey and cheese curds.

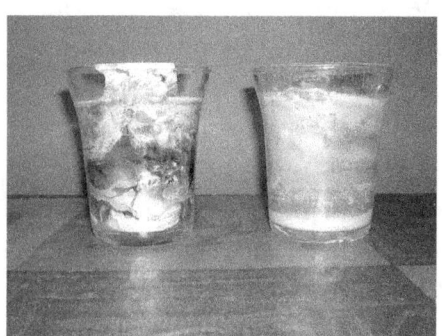 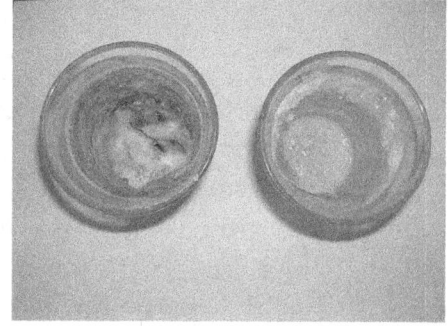

Close to two months later, the liquids have evaporated almost entirely from both glasses. What remains from the pasteurized milk is greenish/blackish 'rot'. The solids remaining from the raw goat's milk is a dry yellowish cheese.

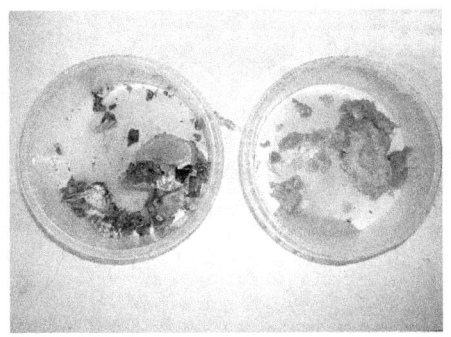
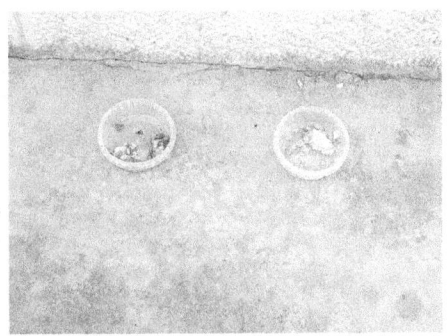

The solids are transferred to plastic bowls – bring on the cats!

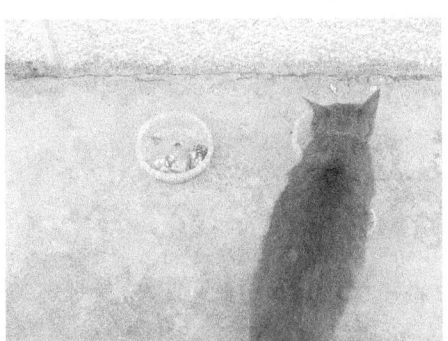
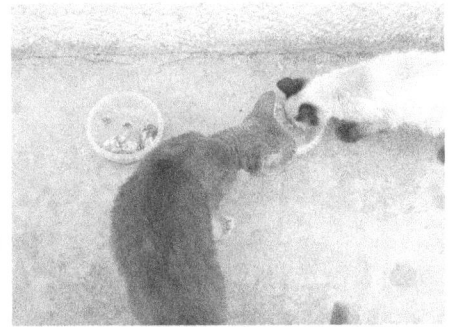

First to arrive is Gray…and one by one the 'word gets out'.

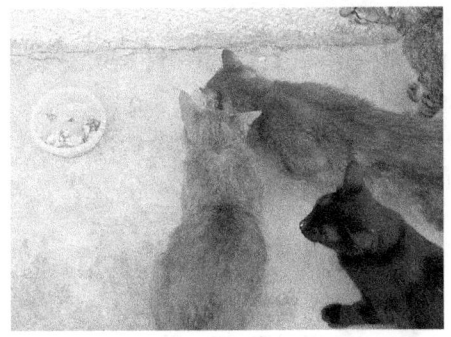
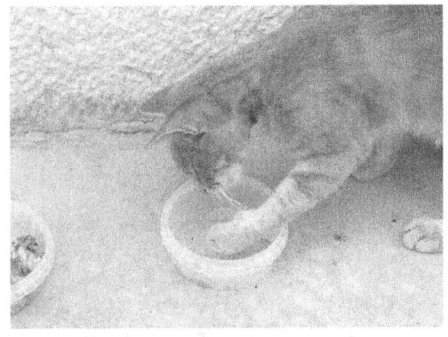

Nivi finally makes it (upper right)

Gray – finger lickin' good!

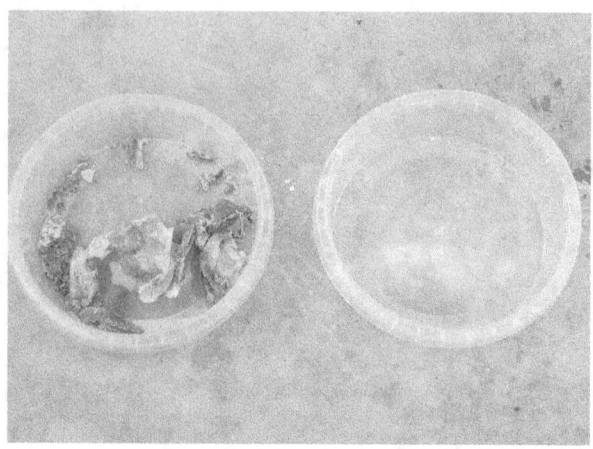

The bowl with the two-month old cheese from raw goat's milk has been licked clean. The green-black pasteurized rot remained untouched!

Why pasteurize in the first place?

Research overwhelmingly demonstrates that pasteurization creates higher rates of degenerative illnesses in both humans and in animal research.[48] For all of its heath detriments, why has pasteurization become the norm over the last 100 years? Shortly after the start of the twentieth century, the sloppy production methods, delivery through streets laden with fly infested horse manure, and lack of hygienic cool storage areas in many homes (later known as refrigerators) did result in the contamination of the raw milk. Drinking of the milk did cause a considerable amount of disease and death.

Pasteurization supplied a practical and economic solution to the ultimately disease-infected milk. It was necessary to prevent the spread of communicable disease. There was no simple way to enforce hygiene on so many small independent milk-producing farms, and then guarantee its safe delivery to the end user. As a result, the monster had overcome the creator. Once considered a wonder treatment (before pasteurization), medical literature today no longer advocates the use of raw milk diets[49] as a universal way to cure disease.

Raw milk cures have gone the route of the phonograph record and the manual typewriter. Pasteurized milk, however, is not used today to cure anything.

Epidemics and pasteurized milk

The proponents of pasteurization would have us believe that epidemics caused by milk became extinct with the widespread use of pasteurization. The U.S. government has documented numerous outbreaks of food-borne illness from pasteurized milk.[50]

1945	1,492 cases for the year in the U.S.
1945	One outbreak, 300 cases in Phoenix, Arizona
1945	Several outbreaks, 468 cases of gastroenteritis, nine deaths, in Great Bend, Kansas
1976	Outbreak of Yersinia enterocolitica in 36 children, 16 of them had appendectomies due to pasteurized chocolate milk
1978	One outbreak, 68 cases in Arizona
1982	Over 17,000 cases of Yersinia enterocolitica in Memphis, TN
1982	172 cases, with over 100 hospitalized from a three-Southern-state area
1983	One outbreak, 49 cases of Listeriosis in Massachusetts
1984	August, One outbreak S. typhimurium, approximately 200 cases, at one plant in Melrose Park, IL

1984	November, One outbreak S. typhimurium, at same plant in Melrose Park, IL
1985	March, One outbreak, 16,284 confirmed cases, at same plant in Melrose Park, IL
1985	197,000 cases of antimicrobial-resistant Salmonella infections from one dairy in California
1985	1,500+ cases, Salmonella culture confirmed in Northern Illinois
1987	Massive outbreak of over 16,000 culture-confirmed cases of antimicrobial-resistant Salmonella typhimurium traced to pasteurized milk in Georgia
1993	Two outbreaks statewide, 28 cases Salmonella infection
1994	Three outbreaks, 105 cases, E. Coli & Listeria in California
1993-1994	Outbreak of Salmonella enteritidis in over 200 due to pasteurized ice cream in Minnesota, South Dakota and Wisconsin
1995	1 outbreak, 3 cases in California
1995	Outbreak of Yersinia enterocolitica in ten children, three hospitalized due to post-pasteurization contamination
1996	Two outbreaks Campylobactor and Salmonella, 48 cases in California
1997	Two outbreaks, 28 cases Salmonella in California

Pasteurization is also not a magic wand able to neutralize harmful ingredients that find their way into the cows' commercial food sources. Ultimately they find their way into the milk supply...through pasteurization...to the dining room table.

The 1973 Michigan PBB (polybromylated biphenyl) disaster[51] is proof of this. PBBs are manmade chemicals that were used as fire retardants in plastics. At the time, one of the plants manufacturing PBB was the Michigan Chemical Company. The same St. Louis, Michigan plant also manufactured a magnesium oxide cattle feed supplement. According to the State of Michigan Department of Community Health, in 1973, 10 to 20 50-pound bags of PBB were accidentally sent to the Michigan Farm Bureau Service instead of the cattle feed supplement. Other sources are less conservative regarding the actual amount of PBB that made its way into cattle feed.

Five years after the contamination, about 97% of Michigan's residents showed measurable levels of the chemical. In August 1976, the Department of Public Health found that 22 of 26 samples of human breast milk from the general population in Michigan showed the presence of PBB. Later, a more scientific study detected PBB in the breast milk of 95% of nursing mothers tested in Michigan's Lower Peninsula.[52]

This is the real catastrophe of this disaster. Children who weren't even born at the time of the disaster have likely been exposed. The possible long-term health consequences remain a point of concern and uncertainty. There is no medical treatment that will lower PBB levels in the human body. Daniel Rosen from the Centers for Disease Control (CDC) in Atlanta, GA published a 1995 article in Environmental Health Perspectives citing approximately 10.8 years as the calculated half-life of PBBs within the human body.

Although not easy to calculate specific consequences due to specific amounts of human exposure to PBBs through diet, the following problems have been reported and seem to be associated with this PBB exposure:

- Musculoskeletal problems, especially joint disorders (pain, swelling, and crepitation)
- Neurological symptoms (tiredness, fatigue, headaches, dizziness, and unusually long sleep hours)
- Evidence of higher liver function
- Immunological abnormalities (decreased number of circulating lymphocytes and altered responses to tests of the functional integrity of these cells)
- Elevated levels of spontaneous abortion rates among second-generation Michigan women born after the 1973 incident
- Increased risk of cancers of the breast, the digestive system and for lymphoma
- Shorter menstrual cycle and with a longer bleed time during menstruation.

Since the late 1970's, the Michigan Department of Community Health has been keeping tabs on approximately 4,000 people, mainly families and neighbors on farms who consumed the most contaminated products, and their offspring.

Incidentally, milk products (pasteurized) and beef (cooked) were not the only products affected. Feed for other animals was contaminated when it was mixed using the same machinery; carcasses of cattle not fit for sale were rendered to yield protein supplements in other animal feed. By the end of 1975, as a result of the PBB contamination, about 28,900 cattle, 5,920 pigs, and 1.5 million chickens had been destroyed. Eight hundred and sixty-five tons of contaminated animal feed were buried around the state. In addition, 17,940 lb of cheese, 2,630 lb of butter, 34,000 lb of dry milk products, and nearly five million eggs were also destroyed.

The moral of this story: In addition to the inherent disadvantages that pasteurization causes, it also does not guarantee that the final product will be free of harmful additives.

Pasteurization is not the only problem...

Proud family-run dairy farms are quickly becoming a thing of the past. Once upon a time, dairy cows would roam the pastures, eating fresh grass to their hearts' content. Many dairy cows today are confined to small, contained areas with no grass, no sunshine, no roaming around. There were over 3.7 million dairy farms in the U.S. in 1950. By the year 2000 the number had dwindled to slightly over 105,000.[53] Some of the larger confinement farms contain thousands of cows. More than half of all the milk production today in the U.S. comes from operations containing over 500 cows.

The cows themselves have become high-production milk machines. In 1950 the average output per dairy cow was slightly less than two gallons of milk per day. Cows fed a diet high in grains and growth hormones yield over six gallons per day.[54] The high incidence of disease in cows kept in confinement facilities also results in the widespread use of antibiotics, many which are resistant to prolonged heating.[55] Nutritionally, who cares? It makes sense economically -- even to the extent that the average lifespan of today's confinement dairy cow is only 42 months; cows on pasture live 12 to 15 years.

No, cows are not cats. Also, people are not cats. However, the observations made by Dr. Pottenger (chapter 4) regarding the milk from grass-fed cows as opposed to grain-fed cows on his cats should be of great concern to us humans. Grain-fed cattle also tend to have a more acidic intestine which is more conducive to harboring pathogenic bacteria than cattle fed mostly grass and hay. Grain-fed cattle were found to have a one million-fold more acid-resistant E.coli than cattle fed hay.[56] In the previous chart, you will notice E.coli contamination was found in pasteurized milk in 1994 in California.

It is almost ironic that because many cows kept in confinement conditions are overly sick and produce inferior milk, the way to insure that this inferior milk is 'safe' for human consumption is to pasteurize it![57]

Today there is a solution for the big city dweller wanting to drink healthy raw milk. It is called certified raw milk. The term 'certified' means that the milk is inspected by a board of physicians and is certified by them to meet rigid standards of cleanliness. The cows are regularly checked and must be in PERFECT health. Before milking, they are meticulously cleaned. The workers themselves with access to a certified raw milk facility must also be in perfect health and keep themselves meticulously clean. Personal habits are under constant supervision. Frequent and regular bacterial testing insures that the milk is of the highest quality.[58]

Whole books could be written on the history and all the other aspects of raw vs. pasteurized milk in our daily diet, including politics and government meddling. In fact, they already have been! My favorites are

The Untold Story of Milk by Dr. Ron Schmid, New Trends Publishing

And

The Milk Book by Dr. William Campbell Douglass II, Rhino Publishing

Both are recommended, and no, they are by no means identical. For example, they take opposite sides on the 'homogenization' issue; i.e. is homogenization of milk a cause of heart disease?[59]

To keep abreast of what is relevant and important regarding 'real milk', visit the Real Milk Campaign of the Weston A. Price Foundation at http://www.realmilk.com.

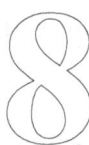

Two Postulates

A postulate is a hypothesis advanced as an essential
presupposition, condition, or premise
of a train of reasoning.
Merriam-Webster Dictionary

Wikipedia defines a postulate as "a statement or assumption that is agreed by everyone to be so obvious or self-evident that no proof is necessary, and which can be used to prove other statements or theorems." Simply stated, a postulate is G-d given. Period.

In junior high geometry class, we memorized geometry Postulate #1: For any two points, there is exactly one line containing them. From this postulate, we could then prove the following theorem: Two lines intersect in at most one point.

Many things in our lives are governed by this same analogy. There is the self-evident base, on which further statements or 'theorems' are derived.

Under author's notes at the beginning of this book, I stated

"This book starts out under the premise that cholesterol and saturated fat are not the causes of heart disease. Period. End of story."

I began believing this premise when writing SASHA and since its publication, I accept it lock, stock and barrel. Stated in different terminology:

<u>Postulate</u>
Saturated Fat and Cholesterol do
not cause heart disease.

On this assumption, I can substantiate a theorem that foods containing saturated fat and cholesterol are not harmful to my cardiovascular system. According to this argument, I could eat anything without regard to saturated fat and cholesterol content, and I would not be harming my health. This would include of course, among other things, the whole spectrum of dairy products available in any supermarket, right? What then is logically wrong with this argument as stated?

A postulate cannot be wrong by definition. It is, after all, a postulate, an axiom. I am convinced that pasteurized dairy products with the natural nutriments and enzymes missing do have a definite place in the myriad of health problems plaguing the Western world today, heart disease among them. Something is wrong with the theorem; therefore there must be something lacking in the postulate.

The type and form of the saturated fat/cholesterol that most people consume does not fit the postulate! Dr. Howell stated that when commercial fat deprived of its lipase companion confronts hydrochloric acid in the stomach, it faces a harsh experience and may be improperly metabolized when it reaches body tissues later.[60]

Conclusion: the theorem 'foods containing saturated fat and cholesterol are not harmful to my cardiovascular system' is not entirely valid so therefore cannot be automatically derived from Postulate #1 as stated. We will need to use an additional postulate and modify the first postulate to be correct in all cases.

Postulate 2
Saturated fat and cholesterol from processed/heated foods **can** cause heart disease.

Modification of Postulate 1:

Postulate 1
Saturated fat and cholesterol from raw unprocessed foods **do not** cause heart disease.

The irony of it all is that my cardiologist and all the other doctors still advocating the validity of the lipid hypothesis have been saying all along that saturated fat and cholesterol cause heart disease. Two very similar sounding postulates. Two very different consequences. So similar, but so different.

9

A Very Thin Chapter on Fats

The first law of dietetics seems to be:
if it tastes good, it's bad for you.
Isaac Asimov

The polyunsaturated fats paradox, or is it?

For decades the anti-saturated fat and anti-cholesterol campaign has been accompanied by the pro-polyunsaturated fat agenda. As recently as August 2003, the USDA was still carrying the polyunsaturated heart healthy banner 'polyunsaturated fatty acids have been linked to lower incidences of heart disease'.[61] This particular article did later mention the dark sides of polyunsaturated fats, i.e. lacking strong stability traits and being prone to oxidation, however, it did seem to stress the positive 'lower incidences of heart disease'.

Here in Israel, we have the dubious distinction of having one of the highest dietary polyunsaturated/saturated fat ratios in the world. We consume 8% more omega-6 polyunsaturated fatty acids than in the USA, and 10-12% higher than in most European countries. According to USDA guidelines we should be heart disease free. Instead we suffer from a high prevalence of cardiovascular diseases and hypertension. This was published in an article entitled *Diet and disease--the Israeli paradox: possible dangers of a high omega-6 polyunsaturated fatty acid diet.*[62]

What drew my attention to this article was a key word in the title 'paradox'. Merriam-Webster gives several definitions for the word 'paradox':

> *a statement that is seemingly contradictory or opposed to common sense and yet is perhaps true*

and also

> *an argument that apparently derives self-contradictory conclusions by valid deduction from acceptable premises*

Wikipedia states:

> *A paradox is an apparently true statement or group of statements that leads to a contradiction or a situation which defies intuition.*

The bottom line: there is no paradox here. As we shall see, the quantity and quality of the polyunsaturated fats in the Western diet is neither heart friendly or healthy.

Plaque rupture

Plaque rupture (rupture of scar tissue covering an atheroma – chapter 10) is a major trigger of acute coronary events. Sixty to seventy percent of acute coronary syndromes evolve from mildly to moderately obstructive atherosclerotic plaques.[63] The promoters of the prevalent lipid hypothesis would have us believe that aortic plaque formation is caused by eating cholesterol and saturated fat.

Atherosclerotic plaques contain a disproportionately high concentration of the omega-6 fatty acid linoleic acid; plaque content of linoleic acid correlates with dietary intake, in particular **polyunsaturated vegetable oils**. Higher plaque concentrations of linoleic acid are also associated with an increased likelihood of plaque rupture.[64]

What is the connection between saturated fats, poly-unsaturated fat and plaque formation? In 1994, Dr. Carl V. Felton et al summarized this quite nicely:

> *No associations were found with saturated fatty acids. These findings imply a direct influence of dietary polyunsaturated fatty acids on aortic plaque formation and suggest that **current trends favouring increased intake of polyunsaturated fatty acids should be reconsidered**.*[65] (Bold emphasis is mine.)

These findings were confirmed again in 2001 in a later study.[66]

Essential Fatty Acids

In SASHA I discussed the importance of steering clear of all partially hydrogenated oils and the resulting trans-fat. This is only the beginning.

Essential Fatty Acids (EFAs) are fats the body absolutely needs but does not have the ability to produce; hence the term 'essential'. Therefore, they must be obtained from the diet. The body needs only **small quantities** of EFAs for normal functioning.[67]

EFAs allow the entry into cells of important nutrients as well as the removal of toxins from the cells. In addition, EFAs are converted to substances that affect cell growth, platelet aggregation (blood clotting ability) and blood pressure, subjects of prime importance to cardiovascular health.

We have all heard of omega-3 and omega-6 fats. These are both EFAs and belong to the polyunsaturated family of fats. EFAs are used to make two classes of hormone like substances known as the prostaglandins. Prostaglandins derived from omega-6 EFAs (prostaglandin-1) typically stimulate the immune system (coagulation) and help form blood clots. Prostaglandins derived from omega-3 (prostaglandin-3) EFAs typically down regulate the immune response to maintain blood fluidity.

Our ancestors consumed a diet with a 1:1 – 3:1 balance[68] between the omega-6 and omega-3 essential fatty acids. It is speculated that in today's Western society the ratio of omega-6/omega-3 fatty acids may be as high as 20:1 - 30:1.[69] Excessive amounts of omega-6 polyunsaturated fatty acids and a very high omega-6/omega-3 ratio promotes the pathogenesis of many diseases, including cardiovascular and inflammatory disease; a lower omega-6/omega-3 ratio exerts suppressive effects.[70]

EFAs, which are polyunsaturated fats, are vitally essential for human health; on the other hand, we see that accumulated plaque in our arteries and the resulting heart disease is polyunsaturated fat intensive.

Is it only a wrong balance of omega-6/omega-3 that is causing the accumulation of the polyunsaturated junk in our arteries? Modern medicine has found a simple solution for today's omega-6/omega-3 imbalance – we should all consume more omega-3 rich foods, such as fish oil supplements. History has taught us that easy one-sided solutions can often be counterproductive, if not outright dangerous.

The last two generations were weaned on the theory that HDL is 'good' cholesterol and LDL is 'bad' cholesterol; basically we were taught that fat in general is bad. Two decades of statins to lower LDL and fats in the blood to prevent heart disease did indeed lower LDL levels, but did not curb the heart disease epidemic.

The last two generations were taught that salt is 'unnecessary' – it causes high blood pressure. Supermarkets today even sell salt-free salt substitutes. It wasn't until professional athletes started suffering (even dying) from hyponatremia (low concentration of sodium in the blood) that the importance of proper salt intake was accepted.

We all 'know' that as far as breathing is concerned, oxygen is 'good' and carbon dioxide (CO_2) is 'bad'. We inhale the good and exhale the bad. Dr. Konstantin Buteyko has demonstrated that there must be enough carbon dioxide in our systems for the oxygen to circulate effectively; long term over-breathing (hyperventilation) ultimately leads to organ damage and the development of illnesses.[71]

And now the latest fad, unmonitored omega-3 supplementation to correct our imbalance.

Basic View of Polyunsaturated Fatty Acids (PUFA)

Omega-3	Omega-6
Alpha-Linolenic Acid (ALA) *	Linoleic Acid (LA) *
Eicosapentaenoic acid (EPA) **	Arachidonic Acid (AA) **
Docosahexaenoicacid (DHA) **	Gamma Linolenic Acid (GLA)**
* Essential Fatty Acid ** Conditional Fatty Acid	

There are three major forms of omega-3 EFAs that are contained in the foods we eat that are used by the body: alpha-linolenic acid (ALA), eicosapentaenoic acid (EPA), and docosahexaenoic acid (DHA). Once eaten, the body can convert some of the ALA to EPA and DHA, although in small quantities (DHA in very small quantities). Higher omega-6 to omega-3 ratios in the diet reduces this conversion further.[72] Not everyone is capable of converting some ALA to EPA and DHA. For this reason, EPA and DHA are known as conditional essential fatty acids.

Fatty fishes supply EPA and DHA. The human brain has a high requirement for DHA. Low DHA levels have been linked to low brain serotonin levels.[73]

No doubt, obtaining enough omega-3 is important.

The main omega-6 fatty acids are linoleic acid (LA) and arachadonic Acid (AA). The body normally makes AA from LA. It is also found in animal foods (animal fats and dairy). The body can also produce GLA from LA; however, trans-fatty acids and over consumption of sugar and alcohol inhibit the production of GLA.[74]

Stating that omega-6 causes blood coagulation while omega-3 maintains blood fluidity is oversimplifying the way our body works, and the interaction between processes. AA just happens to be the precursor to prostacyclin, the most potent anti-aggretory agent[75] (a natural blood thinner). Omega-3 and omega-6 eicosanoids* work together in a complementary manner. There is a synergistic effect of omega-3 and omega-6 at low doses which is greater than the effect of high dose of omega-3 alone.[76]

Yes, adequate omega-3 intake is important, but to what extent?

The brain and nervous system, comprising 3% of the total body weight, contains a 1:1 ratio of omega-6 to omega-3 tissue composition.[77] Skin, comprising of 4% of total body weight, contains virtually no omega-3.[78] All the fatty acids in skin tissue are composed of omega-6. Organs and other tissues with 9% of total body weight are made up of a 4:1 omega-6 to omega-3 ratio. Body fat accounts for 15-35% (usually) of total body weight and is comprised of a 22:1 omega-6 to omega-3 ratio. Muscle accounting for approximately 50% of body weight contains from 5.5 to 7.5 times more omega-6 than omega-3, depending on the degree of physical condition.[79]

The problem with most of the omega-6 fatty acids that we consume is that they are already harmful even before we consume them! One of the forms of omega-6

---

* Derived from omega-3 or omega-6 fats. They exert complex control over many bodily systems, including inflammatory and blood-thinning functions.

(linoleic acid aka LA) is found in the primary oil added to most processed foods. It is also contained in significant amounts in many of the commonly used home cooking oils such as corn oil, safflower oil, soybean oil, and sunflower oil. The modern processing of the major sources of omega-6 in our diets involves high temperatures and pressure (most vegetable oils) which has hydrogenated them into trans-fats or adulterated them with chemicals and preservatives.

This does extend the shelf life which may be great for all the middlemen along the way; however it is very harmful to the final consumer.

Here we get to the crux of the problem. By simply supplementing our diets with important omega-3 rich fish oil, we are not solving the problem of ingesting defective quantities of omega-6!

Polyunsaturated fats are susceptible to oxidation; it is the oxidation of LDL which gives LDL its bad reputation. Oxidized LDL is a predictor of atherosclerosis and cardiovascular disease.[80] LDL cholesterol by itself is not.

The LDL serves as a mode of transportation; it is the natural transporter of omega-6 and omega-3 into the cells. Consider the case of jet planes (carrier, mode of transportation) and hijackers. A plane itself carries all passengers; it does not differentiate between law-abiding citizens and murderous hijackers. Sure, we could ban all flights in order to fight the threat of hijacking. Does that sound like a logical solution? I think not.

If the EFAs we consume (polyunsaturated fats in vegetable oils) are already damaged and/or become oxidized, then simply lowering the 'mode of transportation' (LDL) to carry less EFAs and supplementing our diets with healthy omega-3 is not really solving the problem. Without elaborating on all the factors that contribute to the oxygenation of LDL, I want to emphasize again that **oxidized** LDL, and not regular LDL is a predictor of atherosclerosis and cardiovascular disease.[81]

Our creator did a magnificent job in creating us -- so many intertwined and interdependent systems. Our bodies are programmed to regulate levels of sodium, calcium and glucose to within certain limits. There must be a very good reason why our bodies were not equipped with any mechanism whatsoever to also regulate levels of cholesterol.

I will finish this chapter with a final word regarding ratios and total amounts. Olive oil, for example, is not polyunsaturated oil; it is monounsaturated oil. It is considered to be healthy oil, and is the basis of the 'Mediterranean diet'.

On the following chart[82] we see that the omega-6 to omega-3 ratio is still considered to be high – even higher than soybean oil.

Oil	Omega-6/Omega-3 Ratio
Sunflower oil	No Omega-3
Safflower oil	202:1
Corn oil	71:1
Olive oil	11:1
Soybean oil	7:1

I want to distinguish between high omega-6 to omega-3 *ratio*, and actual *amount*. In the following charts, the total amount of omega-6 and omega-3 is listed as grams per teaspoon:

Oil	Grams per teaspoon	
	Omega-6	Omega-3
Safflower oil,	10.1	0.05
Corn oil	7.9	0.11
Sunflower oil	8.95	
Soybean oil,	6.95	0.93
Olive oil	1.12	0.1

You may notice that a big advantage to olive oil is that is does not contribute to the overall total body unfavorable omega-6 to omega-3 ratio; its ratio is indeed unfavorable, however, the absolute quantities of both are low. Without getting into a discussion over the virtues of olive oil, it could also be said that olive oil is simply not as bad as the other oils.

We will return to polyunsaturated fats and Essential Fatty Acids in Chapter 18.

10

What's New Since SASHA?

You do not really understand something unless you can explain it to your grandmother.
Albert Einstein

We all know what arteries are. I have mentioned them throughout this book. We visualize them as very small garden hoses; hoses transport water, arteries transport blood. Here the similarity ends. Whereas a garden hose is one thick layer of a single material, an artery is comprised of several different layers and cell types. Of particular importance to us are the cells that line the interior surface of blood vessels, known as 'endothelial cells'. Endothelial cells line the entire circulatory system, from the heart to the smallest capillary. This layer comprised of endothelial cells is known as the 'endothelium'.

Endothelial cells are involved in many aspects of cardiovascular health, such as atherosclerosis, formation of new blood vessels, blood clotting and blood pressure control.

Plaque that accumulates within arteries forms between the endothelium and the outer layers. It does not form on the inner surface of the artery.[83] When the plaque accumulates to the point where it causes a bulge protruding the inner wall into the bloodstream, this bulge is known as an atheroma.

We will encounter endothelial cells/function extensively throughout the rest of this book.

The NIH Golomb Study

It was the NIH study[84] chaired by Prof. Beatrice Golomb regarding the negative side effects caused by statins that alerted me to the source of my dysfunction during my two statin-taking years. Among the complaints she was researching that affected me personally were memory loss, personality changes, irritability, and cognitive problems.

Today, recognition of the adverse effects caused by statins has emerged from underground and is well documented. What I do want to stress are her findings regarding a separate and serious problem suffered by the statin victims. The ignorance and/or denial of the medical community regarding adverse side effects which simply compounds the personal distress and frustration of the statin victim:

> *Patients perceived that physicians failed to appreciate the impact of the statin adverse effects on their quality of life. Statements attributed to physicians by many patients included: denial of*

existence of any statin adverse effects, denial of specific statin adverse effects (muscle, memory, neuropathy), attribution of symptoms to age, attribution of symptoms to "imagination", and dismissal of the importance of symptoms. ..... Subjects' responses suggest that many physicians may be unfamiliar with the spectrum of adverse events even for widely used preventive agents; and that physicians may be perceived to convey a lack of appreciation of the impact of symptoms on patients.[85]

EDTA Chelating Therapy

EDTA Chelating Therapy is not something new; I discussed it briefly in SASHA in 2004. Chelating therapy is very effective for people suffering from heavy metal poisoning; the process removes the excess heavy metals from the body. Its application utilizing the synthetic compound EDTA (ethylenediaminetetraacitic acid) can be utilized to improve the condition of patients suffering from clogged arteries. EDTA therapy itself consists of least 20 (generally) intravenous injections, each injection lasting several hours once or twice per week, given over the course of months. The purpose of the therapy is to 'chelate out' part of the accumulated plaque built up in arteries.

Mainstream cardiology has not embraced EDTA Chelating Therapy as a way to improve patients suffering from a variety of cardiovascular ailments. Cardiologists who are at least familiar with the procedure dismiss the process as not proven, ineffective, and dangerous. As such, it is performed at private, 'alternative' clinics. Mainstream cardiology still prefers angioplasty, PCI (stents) and bypass operations as solutions to arteries suffering from impaired flow.

Is EDTA ineffective and dangerous? "Not so," states Dr. Joel Kauffman. He evaluated dozens of clinical trials and concluded that over 87% of patients who have undergone EDTA Chelating Therapy improved.[86] In addition, no ill effects occurred when the procedure was performed correctly.

Will EDTA Chelating Therapy someday be accepted by mainstream cardiology and not remain underground? The future does look encouraging. In 2003, the National Center for Complementary and Alternative Medicine (NCCAM), a part of NIH, initiated a placebo-controlled, double-blind five-year study involving about 2,000 participants.[87] This study, which will cost approximately $30 million, is over 20 times larger than any previous study of EDTA Chelating Therapy. It is designed to be large enough to detect if there are indeed benefits or risks associated with the therapy.

Aspirin inhibits production of GLA

In the previous chapter I discussed the importance of the Essential Fatty Acids. Aspirin inhibits the enzyme Delta-6 Desaturase,[88] needed for the production of Gamma-Linoleic Acid (GLA) and important anti-inflammatory prostaglandins. GLA is of particular importance to people suffering from heart disease. It is metabolized to Dihomogamma Linlenic Acid (DGLA) which ultimately produces anti-inflammatory eicosanoids.[89] A study published in 1998 concluded that a combination of GLA and EPA polyunsaturated essential fatty acids produced a statistically significant reduction in systolic blood pressure.[90]

GLA is beneficial not only to heart patients. A deficiency in essential fatty acids, including GLA and EPA, can lead to severe bone loss and osteoporosis. Clinical studies have reported that supplements of GLA and EPA help maintain or increase bone mass.[91]

Many women suffer from Premenstrual Syndrome (PMS). PMS is characterized by breast tenderness, feelings of depression, irritability and swelling and bloating due to fluid retention. GLA supplementation proved to be highly effective in the treatment of women suffering from PMS.[92]

Millions of people take aspirin as a preventative measure against having a first heart attack or preventing a second one. I wonder how many of them have been advised to reinforce their diets with GLA. For this large population, GLA is no longer a conditional EFA; it has become an unconditional essential fatty acid, and must be consumed in the diet.

LDL levels and Statins

In 2001, I was advised to make sure my LDL levels stayed below 100. This was the reason why my Pravastatin (statin) dosage was increased from 10mg/day to 20mg/day; my LDL blood levels had surpassed the 100 threshold. For many years, high LDL cholesterol has been the accepted yardstick by family doctors and cardiologists for the off the cuff evaluation that we are in the high-risk category for heart problems.

Statins are *extremely* effective in reducing the blood level of LDL. The standard opening line when sitting across from a cardiologist is 'Let's see those cholesterol stats', and in particular, 'What about the LDL level?'

In 2005, the American Heart Association (AHA) along with the National Heart, Lung, and Blood Institute (NHLBI) published new guidelines[93] regarding recommended acceptable LDL Cholesterol Levels. For people diagnosed as moderate risk, the maximum level of LDL was set at 130mg/dL.

High-risk patients were defined as having established atherosclerotic CVD, diabetes, or ten-year risk for CHD > 20%. The recommended maximum level of LDL for high-risk people was set at 100mg/dL. Very high-risk patients were defined as likely to have major CVD events during the next few years or already had recent acute coronary syndromes or have established CHD in addition to other multiple major risk factors. The recommended maximum level of LDL for very high-risk people was set at 70mg/dL.

Until fairly recently, the cardiology world attributed cardiovascular benefits of statins to their LDL lowering abilities. This in turn strengthened the proponents of the lipid hypothesis. Recent (mid-2006, 2007) research papers appearing in peer reviewed scientific journals are finally acknowledging and stating emphatically that **beneficial cardiovascular effects of statins are independent of their LDL lowering properties**.

Medicine is a science, and changes to prevailing scientific consensus apparently never come easy. Galileo Galilei, known today simply as Galileo, is often referred to as the 'father of modern astronomy', as the 'father of modern physics', and even as the 'father of science'. His support of the Copernican astronomy concept (sun-centered solar system) was considered to be on the border of heresy by the all-powerful Catholic Church during his time. The possible consequences of such actions are obvious.

Sure, you must be thinking -- we are more civilized today then our predecessors of 400 years ago. But are we really? In SASHA I discussed Dr. Kilmer McCully's research, which was not in line with the medical consensus. He concluded that cholesterol, particularly LDL cholesterol, was not a cause of heart disease. His research centered on homocysteine levels and ultimately resulted in his banishment from Harvard University and Massachusetts General Hospital. He was denied a new position for more than two years because of his research.[94]

This change of direction on the part of medical researchers regarding the cholesterol-independent benefits of statins is of such major importance that I will list a number of the works here. Bold emphasis is mine.

- *The benefits observed with statin treatment appear to be greater than what might be expected from reduction in lipid levels alone, suggesting effects beyond cholesterol lowering.* ***These cholesterol-independent effects have been called "pleiotropic".*** *The cholesterol-independent or "pleiotropic" effects of statins involve improvement of endothelial function, stability of atherosclerotic plaques, decrease of oxidative stress and inflammation, and inhibition of thrombogenic response. These pleiotropic effects of statins have been proposed as key properties of these drugs to reduce cardiovascular morbidity and mortality.*[95]

- *..... statins, have been reported to exert actions independent of their lipid-lowering effects....*

*...Cerivastatin reduces monocyte adhesion to vascular endothelium under physiological flow conditions via down regulation of integrin adhesion molecules and inhibition of actin polymerization via RhoA inactivation. Our findings have **important implications for the lipid-independent effects of statins**.*[96]

- *With an increase in use and popularity, a number of beneficial actions of the statins unrelated to their cholesterol-lowering ability have been reported. .... Of central focus in this paper is the **cholesterol-independent benefit** of this group of agents on the cardiovascular system, particularly on the lowering of systemic blood pressure.*[97]

- *Acute coronary syndromes involve a complex interplay between the vessel wall, inflammatory cells, and the coagulation cascade. **Statins possess beneficial effects that are independent of low-density lipoprotein cholesterol lowering** and that have favorable effects on inflammation, the endothelium, and the coagulation cascade. There is now accumulating evidence that these lipid-independent pleiotropic effects are clinically relevant in the management of acute coronary syndromes.*[98]

- *Inflammation contributes importantly to all stages of atherosclerosis, including the onset of acute thrombotic complications. ...... Moreover, **statins have been shown to possess several pleiotropic properties independent of cholesterol lowering** in experimental settings.*[99]

- *Statins decrease mortality in patients with coronary artery disease. However, chronic heart failure (CHF) patients were often excluded in such trials. Statins possess pharmacologic properties **(independent of cholesterol lowering) that may be beneficial on ventricular remodeling** in such patients.*[100]

- *Macrophage cyclooxygenase-2 (COX-2) plays an important role in prostaglandin E2 and thromboxane A2 production. Statins are inhibitors of HMG CoA (3-Hydroxy-3-methylglutaryl coenzyme A) reductases and cholesterol synthesis, which block the expression of several inflammatory proteins **independent of their capacity to lower endogenous cholesterol.***[101]

- *Accelerated coronary arteriosclerosis remains a major problem for the long-term survival of cardiac transplant recipients……. HMG-CoA reductase inhibitors, or statins, are widely prescribed to lower plasma cholesterol level. Accumulating evidence indicates **that statins have various effects on vascular cells which are independent of their lipid-lowering effect.***[102]

- *Statins, the most widely prescribed cholesterol-lowering drugs, are considered to be first-line therapeutics for the prevention of coronary heart disease and atherosclerosis………This article summarizes these **cholesterol-lowering-independent effects of statins**, termed "pleiotropic effects", and the underlying mechanisms, as well as the preclinical* *experimental approaches that would be useful to evaluate the effects of statins.* [103]

- *3-Hydroxy-3-methylglutaryl coenzyme A (HMG-CoA) reductase inhibitors* **(statins) exhibit a wide variety of anti-atherogenic* effects that may be independent of their property to lower plasma cholesterol.** .... *The present findings suggest that statin-mediated immunomodulation by inhibiting MIP-1alpha could contribute to the beneficial effects of statin therapy independent of lowering plasma cholesterol.* [104]

- *Statins are effective drugs in the prevention of cardiovascular disease. Recent studies suggested that* **statins have additional beneficial effects on the vascular wall independent of their cholesterol-lowering effects.** .... *The finding that atorvastatin inhibited ACE upregulation may represent a novel pleiotropic action and an additional beneficial effect of statins in treatment of cardiovascular disease.* [105]

- *Support for pleiotropic effects of statins in these trials has been provided not only by these acute effects but also by apparent differences in efficacy between various statin regimens that seem unrelated to their effects on serum cholesterol levels........ This article reviews some of the key statin trials in ACS and assesses the evidence for benefits of these* **drugs independent of their effects on LDL cholesterol.** [106]

---

* Fatty degeneration of the inner coat of the arteries, an abnormal fatty deposit in an artery

- *Statins are the 3-hydroxy-3-methylglutaryl coenzyme A reductase inhibitors that function as potent inhibitors of cholesterol biosynthesis and have been used for many years for the treatment of hypercholesterolemia. However, accumulating experimental and clinical studies have revealed that the **health benefits associated with statins treatment, particularly those conferred on the cardiovascular system**, **were the cholesterol-independent**[107]*

- *Inflammation plays a key role in progression and destabilization of atherosclerotic plaque. 18F-fluorodeoxyglucose PET is a promising tool for visualizing inflammation of atherosclerotic plaque. Antiinflammatory action is one of **the pleiotropic effects of statins**. .... 18F-fluorodeoxyglucose PET visualized plaque inflammation and simvastatin attenuated it. The **LDL-C-independent effects** of simvastatin may participate in the beneficial effect.[108]*

- *Recently, it has been reported that 3-hydroxy-3-methylglutaryl coenzyme A (HMG-CoA) reductase **inhibitors (statins) exhibit vasoprotective effects, which are independent of their cholesterol-lowering effects**.[109]*

- *Statins inhibit cholesterol synthesis and produce pleiotropic, **cholesterol-independent effects including endothelial NO synthase** (eNOS) stimulation and increased expression.[110]*

- ***Statins produce cholesterol-independent, anti-inflammatory effects**, which result at least in*

86

part from increased endothelial nitric oxide production[111]

- *The 3-hydroxy-3-methyl-glutaryl coenzyme A (HMG-CoA) reductase inhibitors are widely prescribed for hyperlipidemia, but they also **exhibit anti-inflammatory actions that appear to be independent of their suppressive actions on plasma cholesterol levels**.*[112]

- *Besides the action on plasma lipid levels, statins show a series of ancillary effects defined as all of their **vascular and nonvascular effects independent from the cholesterol reduction**.*[113]

- *Subgroup analyses of large clinical trials, however, have suggested that the beneficial effects of statins may extend to mechanisms beyond cholesterol reduction. Indeed, recent experimental and clinical evidence indicates that some of the **cholesterol-independent or "pleiotropic" effects of statins** may be mediated through improving or restoring endothelial function, enhancing the stability of atherosclerotic plaques, and decreasing oxidative stress and vascular inflammation.*[114]

In the beginning of this section I discussed the AHA and NHLBI recommendation for maximum LDL level of 130mg/dL for people at only 'moderate risk' and 70mg/dL for 'very high risk'.

- *Recent national recommendations have proposed that physicians should titrate lipid therapy to achieve low-density lipoprotein (LDL) cholesterol* *levels less than 1.81 mmol/L (<70mg/dL) for patients at very high cardiovascular risk and less than 2.59 mmol/L (<100mg/dL) for patients at high cardiovascular risk. .... For those with LDL cholesterol levels less than 3.36 mmol/L (<130mg/dL), the authors found no clinical trial subgroup analyses or valid cohort or case-control analyses suggesting that the degree to which LDL cholesterol responds to a statin independently predicts the degree of cardiovascular risk reduction. .... Clear, compelling evidence supports near-universal empirical statin therapy in patients at high cardiovascular risk (regardless of their natural LDL cholesterol values), **but current clinical evidence does not demonstrate that titrating lipid therapy to achieve proposed low LDL cholesterol levels is beneficial or safe.**[115]*

.

- *Therefore, we could find no experimental evidence suggesting that the degree of LDL cholesterol reduction is an independent predictor of cardiovascular risk if LDL cholesterol level is less than 3.36 mmol/L (<130 mg/dL)........In this review, we found no high-quality clinical evidence to support currently proposed treatment goals for LDL cholesterol...... **We could find no published high-quality clinical evidence supporting titration of lipid therapy based on proposed LDL cholesterol targets.**[116]*

Statins do indeed reduce LDL levels. So what? LDL levels do not cause heart disease. I adapted this agenda as a way of life when writing SASHA. Statins do have beneficial effects for people with heart disease. Does this mean I am like many mainstream cardiologists who ponder 'Should statins, like fluoride, be added to our drinking water?'[117] Anyone who has read SASHA can guess what my answer to that would be. We will return to the statin discussion shortly.

Torcetrapib

Since Dr. Ancel Keys' 1953 so-called proof[118] that fat intake was the cause of death from coronary heart disease in his infamous 'six-country study', the cardiologic world has been searching for ways to lower fat and blood cholesterol, particularly the 'bad' LDL. Why did I label his study as 'infamous'? Dr. Keys actually had access to, and ignored, the data from an additional 16 countries; tabulation of data from all 22 countries would have confirmed that his six-country study proved nothing.[119]

Statins, which have been with us for two decades are extremely effective in reducing the level of 'bad' LDL; yet cardiovascular disease, remains the biggest cause of death in the United States. According to the American Heart Association, in every year since 1900 except 1918, CVD accounted for more deaths than any other single cause or group of causes of death in the United States.[120]

Why is mainstream cardiology unsuccessful in preventing so many deaths due to cardiovascular causes? Apparently, another 'trick' was necessary in addition to simply lowering the 'bad' LDL. Pfizer, the maker of Lipitor (LDL lowering statin), the world's best selling medication, came up with an idea of pulling an additional magic rabbit out of the pharmaceutical hat. This new rabbit -- a drug intended to increase levels of the 'good' HDL.

Pfizer was destined to become the savior of all those worried about cardiovascular diseases by supplying us with Lipitor to reduce the LDL, and a new drug which it started developing in the early 1990's named torcetrapib to raise the HDL. We would all become cardiovascular supermen!

The cardiology world was excited about the potential of this latest development. In February 2006, a leading Spanish pharmaceutical journal jumped on the bandwagon and had this to say about torcetrapib.

> *Torcetrapib, a CETP inhibitor, has been shown to be effective, safe and well tolerated when used in combination with atorvastatin therapy. Torcetrapib has been shown to increase HDL cholesterol levels by 46% when given alone and by 61% when given in combination with atorvastatin, as well as to decrease LDL cholesterol levels by more than that achieved by atorvastatin alone. When the dosage of torcetrapib was doubled (at maximum tolerated dose), HDL increased by over 100%. Combination therapy appeared safe and well tolerated.*[121]

(Atorvastatin is the generic name for Lipitor)

And then the bubble burst!

"Doctors leading a global war on heart disease say they are *devastated* by the loss of a new drug they had expected to be an important weapon in the fight against high cholesterol."[122] This is how USA TODAY conveyed the feeling of mainstream cardiologists upon Pfizer's discontinuation of its new HDL increasing wonder drug torcetrapib. Pfizer had hoped to receive final FDA approval to market torcetrapib in the second half of 2007. MSNBC news used similar terms in its description, 'The news is *devastating* to Pfizer...'[123]

Merriam-Webster gives two main definitions for the word 'devastate':

- as to bring to ruin or desolation by violent action
- to reduce to chaos, disorder, or helplessness

According to USA TODAY one might think that doctors are no longer capable of functioning after the Pfizer announcement; according to MSNBC, one might think that Pfizer was forced into bankruptcy. Although Pfizer's stocks may have taken a bit of a beating, Pfizer, which has over 100,000 employees, annual sales of $50 billion and a $7 billion annual research budget,[124] is far from going under.

Pfizer's decision to scrap the torcetrapib project was not a pleasant decision. Since the early 1990's, it had invested close to $1,000,000,000 in torcetrapib's development. That is one billion dollars down the drain! One billion dollars can buy 50,000 brand new Ford Mustangs or over 330 million gallons of gasoline. That is one huge investment to scrap.

A late phase of a large-scale clinical trial that Pfizer hoped would prove the effectiveness and safety of the new drug was not yielding the results Pfizer hoped for. An independent board monitoring the torcetrapib trial counted 82 deaths among the patients who took the drug and 51 deaths in the group who did not take the drug.

The board called on Pfizer to halt the trial. Pfizer agreed and promptly notified the FDA and doctors who had been giving their patients the drug.[125] In addition to the 31 more deaths among the people taking torcetrapib, other discrepancies were seen in a number of patients suffering heart failure and other problems.

Two studies published during the first months of 2007 had this to say about torcetrapib:

- *In patients with familial hypercholesterolemia, the use of torcetrapib with atorvastatin, as compared with atorvastatin alone, did not result in further reduction of progression of atherosclerosis, as assessed by a combined measure of carotid arterial-wall thickness, and was associated with progression of disease in the common carotid segment. These effects occurred despite a large increase in HDL cholesterol levels and a substantial decrease in levels of LDL cholesterol and triglycerides.[126]*

- *The CETP inhibitor torcetrapib was associated with a substantial increase in HDL cholesterol and decrease in LDL cholesterol. It was also associated with an increase in blood pressure, and there was no significant decrease in the progression of coronary atherosclerosis.[127]*

Doctors are **devastated**, Pfizer is **devastated**, but what about those 82 families who hoped that torcetrapib would be the redeemer of their loved ones? These are the people who have the right to feel **devastated**.

Undoubtedly they all signed waivers before the trial confirming that they understood the risks they faced when taking experimental medicines in clinical trials. It is not easy to refuse when being asked by a doctor, who likely saved your life, to participate in a study of this type.

In 2001, while still hospitalized, I also 'agreed' to participate in the now defunct Princess study. The drug that was on trial at the time was a statin called 'Baycol' (cerivastatin). Very shortly after I started taking my daily dosage (at the time I had no way of knowing if I was taking the actual Baycol or a placebo), the project was halted worldwide because of similar reasons -- too many deaths.

Regarding those unfortunate 82 who died while taking torcetrapib, it is of little condolence that due to their low LDL and high HDL levels, they died 'healthy'.

Stents

The implantation of the stent is known medically as PCI (Percutaneous Coronary Intervention). The development of this process was an incredible achievement of technology. Just think about it. Someone arrives to the emergency room in the midst of a heart attack. After stabilizing the condition with proper medication, blood thinners, clot dissolvers, blood vessel expanding medication and the like, a blockage is identified by an angiogram, angioplasty (ballooning) is performed, and a stent is implanted (PCI) in the problem area. Next morning, the patient is on his feet; and within another day or two back to a normal routine.

The nightmare of cardiologists performing stent insertion is the eventual blockage of the stent, a process known as 'restenosis'. Restenosis literally means the reoccurrence of stenosis, which is an abnormal narrowing in a blood vessel.

After the insertion of the standard bare-metal stent, the lining layer of the blood artery starts covering the exposed metal of the stent. This natural procedure takes about a month or so to occur. This is also the reason that I was prescribed the prescription drug Plavix for the first month after my stent insertion in 2001. Together with the aspirin, Plavix is a blood thinner that helps prevent the sticking of foreign objects to the exposed bare-metal stent during that first month.

Classic restenosis is caused by a blood clot (thrombosis), at the sight of treatment or by the gradual growth of abnormal cells within the stent. In many cases, stenting is not a permanent solution, having to be done over in one to four years.[128] Medical science did find a solution for the problem of restenosis occurring in the first months after stenting caused by the growth of abnormal cells within the stent. The solution: a coated drug-eluding stent that indeed lowered the incidence of restenosis during the months following angioplasty.

A drug-eluding stent is a bare-metal stent coated with a special drug that is released from the stent over a period of time. The two leading suppliers of the newer drug-eluding stents are Johnson & Johnson and Boston Scientific. Johnson & Johnson's CYPHER® sirolimus-eluding stent received FDA approval to market in 2003. Boston Scientific's TAXUS® Express2™ paclitaxel-eluding stent entered the market in 2004.

It had seemed that medical technology had found the next generation heir to the bypass operation. The excitement, as history will show, was short-lived. Barely a year had gone by since the introduction of the drug-eluding stents and The Lancet published an article regarding the consequences of discontinuation of blood thinning medications to four stent recipients about a year after their angioplasty. The four, in a very short period of time, suffered a recurring MI (heart attack).[129]

The drug-eluding (coated) stents initially prevent restenosis by inhibiting abnormal cell growth within the stent. However, as it turns out, the drugs used to coat these stents also inhibited the growth of endothelial cells that would prevent the bare metal of the stent from being exposed to the blood.

As a result, when anti-platelet[*] medications are stopped, platelets in the bloodstream may be more likely to 'stick' to the stent, and to begin forming a clot that could block blood flow within a very short time.

In September 2006, Boston Scientific acknowledged that they found a statistically significant difference in the rates of late stent thrombosis (blood clots) when comparing its drug-eluding Taxus model with the earlier generation bare-metal stents.[130]

Johnson & Johnson was not in any hurry to jump on the guilt bandwagon. However, two papers submitted the same month at the World Congress of Cardiology in Barcelona by Drs. Eduardo Camenzind and A. Nordmann showed that Johnson & Johnson had nothing to gloat about. Dr. Nordmann observed not only an increased risk of late mortality and non-fatal myocardial infarction with the sirolimus-eluding stents, but also an apparent increase in all cause mortality after two and three years of follow-up.[131]

---

[*] Platelets (thrombocytes) are the cell fragments circulating in the blood that are involved in the formation of blood clots. Dysfunction or low levels of platelets can lead to excessive (uncontrollable) bleeding, while high levels increase the risk of thrombosis.

A 'simple' solution was found to prevent the sudden occurrence of restenosis for those walking around with the drug-coated stents. The solution is to continue taking blood thinning/anti-clotting/anti-platelet medications like Plavix for the rest of your life. Is there a downside to taking Plavix? Possibly. Plavix is a long-lasting drug that does not have a readily available antidote. Once you start taking it, your platelets are basically out of commission for about seven to ten days, the time it takes for your body to get rid of the old platelets and make new ones.

This could be critical if one is seriously injured in an accident, or needs an urgent operation, etc.

An interesting phenomenon occurred in the stock prices for both Johnson & Johnson and Boston Scientific in the beginning of February, 2007. They both took off south bound. The reason: the long-awaited American College of Cardiology convention to be held in New Orleans at the end of March. At the convention Dr. W. Boden reported that many heart patients routinely implanted with stents to open arteries gain no lasting benefit compared with those treated with drugs only.[132]

Dr. Michael Maeng released the results of a study he conducted involving 12,400 patients in Denmark who were randomly given bare metal or drug-coated stents. He found that the rates of blood clots and heart attacks were similar over 15 months; however, over the last three months of that period, an increased risk of blood clotting and heart attack was seen with drug-coated stents.[133]

Due to the concerns over blood clots, the market saturation of the drug-coated variety of stents dropped to approximately 70% of the market, down from 95% a year earlier. It is no wonder that Boston Scientific's and Johnson & Johnson's stock prices reacted as they did.

What does the future hold for stents? At the March 2007 convention, newer technology stents were presented. Abbott presented a totally bioabsorbable drug-eluding stent made of polylactic acid, which is designed to be fully absorbed and slowly metabolized by the coronary artery. Their everolimus-coated stent will release the drug into the artery and then be slowly absorbed over time. The goal is to leave a healed natural vessel behind.

OrbusNeich's innovation for preventing thrombosis and minimizing restenosis is a stent coated with a substance designed to attract stem cell-like cells from the bloodstream to help the artery heal.

Cordis' experimental stent contains an anti-clotting drug that is contained in tiny wells designed to dissolve over time so that after six months or so the device turns into a plain bare-metal stent.

Will these new stents decrease the occurrence of stent restenosis? Only time will tell. For now, Dr. Camenzind, whose September 2006 presentation at the Barcelona World Congress of Cardiology sparked the current controversy over drug-eluding stents, has his own idea. He finds that the original simple balloon angioplasty device that is currently used as a way to inflate stents may now provide a less invasive way of preventing restenosis.[134]

All in all, a stent is not a natural phenomenon that occurs in the body. Lifestyle habits that are beneficial to people without stents could be harmful to people with them. In SASHA I discussed the importance of keeping homocysteine levels within reasonable limits. One of the ways of accomplishing this is increasing folic acid and vitamins B_6 and B_{12} in the diet. However, for those with stent implantations, it is not recommended to take a B_6/B_{12}/Folate supplement. A conflicting study showed that this vitamin combination caused an increased risk of in-stent restenosis.[135]

To stent or not to stent – that is the question. There are basically two situations when stenting (PCI) is performed. The first is the situation when a patient arrives in the hospital in the midst of a heart attack occurring in real time. The stent is implanted to immediately save the life, or at least minimize imminent permanent damage that may be caused by any other delay. This is NOT the scenario that occurs in most situations.

Most people who have a stent implanted are in a state known as 'stable ischemia'. Something somewhere is blocked up to some degree; however, it is not life threatening in the foreseeable future. Stenting in this case is one of possibly alternatives available to improve or correct the existing problem. In this scenario, it is my opinion that implanting or not implanting a stent is one of the more crucial decisions that one may face in a lifetime. It is no less critical than deciding to marry or not, and to whom; to bring children into this world, or not to; to leave an established stable place of work for whatever reason; and any other major personal/family decision.

The procedure itself has become routine. It might not be the most pleasant procedure in the world; however, it certainly is not all that terrible. As previously mentioned, the recovery and return to normal routine happens within a day or two.

The downside of receiving a stent is long term. Restenosis occurring suddenly at any stage has claimed fatalities, or in a more fortunate situation, a bypass operation. One of the tools doctors still use to try to keep the stent open and free flowing at all costs is to artificially lower blood cholesterol levels. This naturally leads to increased dosages of the famed statins -- the more statins, the lower the LDL. Your cardiologist may be happy with the numbers, but how will you still be functioning? In the case of stable ischemia, in my opinion, the use of stents should be considered as a last resort, and not as a standard practice.

Shock Wave Therapy

A new shock wave therapy for the heart has been found to improve the condition of people with heart blockages/damage by increasing blood flow in the affected region. The method, known as Extracorporeal Cardiac Shock Wave Therapy (CSWT) is based upon the 1980's noninvasive therapy to break up kidney stones (Extracorporeal Shock Wave Lithotripsy). The cardiac shock wave generated is a low-level shock wave as compared to the wave generated to break up kidney stones; it is approximately 10% of that used for lithotripsy treatment.

In 2004, pigs treated with shock wave therapy grew more blood vessels than a control group after only four weeks. There was an increase in the regional myocardial blood flow without any adverse effects.[136] A paper presented to the 12th World Congress on Heart Disease in 2005 stated that:

> *We conclude that CSWT is a new, safe and efficient non-invasive therapy for treating chronic ischemia in CAD patents with refractory angina which are ineligible for other interventions.*[137]

An additional study reported the results regarding nine patients with end-stage coronary artery disease. During a typical session they were hit in 20 to 40 different areas of the heart with 200 pulses each. The hits were focused on areas as small as a two-square-millimeter area. In all patients, blood flow increased and symptoms were alleviated, suggesting the growth of new blood vessels.

> *Myocardial perfusion was improved only in the ischemic area treated with the therapy. These beneficial effects persisted for 12 months. No procedural complications or adverse effects were noted. ..... These results indicate that our extracorporeal cardiac shock wave therapy is an effective and non-invasive treatment for end-stage coronary artery disease, although further careful evaluation is needed.*[138]

Yes, the researchers are meanwhile very optimistic, however, as stated, 'further careful evaluation is needed'.

Nearly 16 million Americans are living with coronary heart disease.[139] Despite progress over the past two decades in treating cardiac disease, there is basically no way to fix damaged heart muscle. During heart attacks, tissue is destroyed when blood is temporarily cut off to a section of the heart, and this tissue can never be repaired.

Close to home here at the Technion University in Haifa, beating cardiac tissue has been created in a lab from human embryonic stem cells, leading to the creation of tiny blood vessels within the tissue.[140] The creation of a vascular system in the tissue is critical for its acceptance by the body.

The technique is aimed at helping patients who have cardiac insufficiency due to heart attacks, making possible tissue implantation into a human heart to repair the damage caused by the attack.

11

Green Gold

$a^2 + b^2 = c^2$ where c is the hypotenuse of a
right-angle triangle.
The Pythagorean Theorem

T his theorem is of fundamental importance in Euclidean Geometry. It serves as a basis for the definition of distance between two points. Decades ago in high school I knew at least one proof of this theorem, as did all the other kids in my math class. Little did I know then that almost 40 years later, Mr. Pythagoras's personal eating doctrines would have such a profound effect on my own eating habits.

Most of us today associate Pythagoras with mathematics. He was also a preacher of mystic doctrines and the founder of the mystic, religious and scientific society called Pythagoreans. It is ironic that Pythagoras received his culinary inspiration here in what is modern day Israel, at a site located a short two-hour drive from where I now live.

The famous historian Flavius Josephus claimed Judaism and/or Hebrew religious thought influenced Pythagoras's thinking.[141] This concurred with other reliable sources, among them Hermippus, an Athenian writer, and Porphyry, a Neoplatonist philosopher.[142]

Pythagoras studied with the Essenes[*] on Mount Carmel, located on the outskirts of modern day Haifa.[143] The Essenes were one of three leading Jewish sects mentioned by Josephus as flourishing in the second century B.C.E., the others being the Pharisees and the Sadducees. The Essenes was a mystic, messianic, even apocalyptic sect of Judaism. They led a very humble existence; they wore very simple clothing, were very pacifistic, and possessions were collectively owned. Members of the northern Essene sect were also known as 'Nazarenes'; Jesus, who was raised in Nazareth (located in the upper Galilee – less than a half-hour drive from modern day Mount Carmel), was known as Jesus the Nazarene.

It was at Mount Carmel with the Essenes that Pythagoras learned about live foods. He took this knowledge with him upon his return to Greece. Pythagoras then became a fruitarian (diet consists of raw fruit and seeds only). He used raw food to cure people with poor digestion. This knowledge was later passed down to Socrates and Plato.[144]

---

[*] There was also a southern Essene sect located closer to Jerusalem. The Dead Sea scrolls comprising more than 800 documents were discovered between 1947 and 1956 in eleven caves in and around the ruins of the ancient settlement of Khirbet Qumran, on the northwest shore of the Dead Sea. Scholars believe that most of the Dead Sea Scrolls were produced by the Essenes.

Adapting an eating habit from an ancient practice from a part of the world so steeped in Jewish and early Christian history is definitely very inspirational. Certainly more inspirational than being influenced by some new processed junk food advertised on TV -- don't you think so?

Nearly 2500 years after Pythagoras, a Swiss physician Maximilian Oskar Bircher-Benner, founder of the famed Bircher-Benner Clinic in Zurich, Switzerland, discovered the writings of Pythagoras and began experimenting with live foods. Around the turn of the previous century (1900) he used a balanced diet of raw vegetables and fruit as a means to heal patients at his sanatorium in Zürich. He was enchanted with chlorophyll (a product of photosynthesis in which plants convert sunlight into carbohydrates), and labeled it 'concentrated sun power'.

These plant-units contain everything which the human organism requires, and in the right proportions: enough of the various proteids, a wealth of the best energy givers, the carbohydrates, from which fats can at any time be formed in the organism or the fats themselves; the minerals necessary for life in the excited state and in the right proportion, and accordingly also the vitamins.....No one therefore need wonder any longer that man can amply nourish himself, grow and keep well with these alone, that ox, horse, stag, roe and even the elephant can build up their proteid-rich bodies from grasses, herbs, leaves and blossoms.[145]

Dr. Bircher stated that nature uses chlorophyll as a body cleanser, rebuilder, and neutralizer of toxins.

In 1930, Dr. Hans Fischer won the Nobel Prize for Chemistry[146] for research on red blood cells. During his research he noticed that hemin, a component of the hemoglobin in blood that carries oxygen, is nearly identical to chlorophyll on the molecular level. The significance of chlorophyll being similar to human hemin is great. A study done 80 years ago showed that the animal body is capable of converting chlorophyll to hemoglobin.[147] It is no wonder that one Steve Meyerowitz labeled chlorophyll as the blood of plants.[148] We will return to Steve very shortly.

Hemin is a web of carbon, hydrogen, oxygen and nitrogen atoms grouped around a single atom of iron. Chlorophyll is a similar web of the same atoms, except that its centerpiece is a single atom of magnesium. This should be of special interest to people worried about heart disease, as magnesium deficiency has been shown to correlate with a number of chronic cardiovascular diseases.[149] It was also found that oral magnesium supplementation in patients with Coronary Artery Disease results in a significant improvement in exercise tolerance, quality of life and possibly beneficially alters outcomes in patients with CAD.[150]

Presenting Dr. Ann

For many people already familiar with the health benefits of chlorophyll, Dr. Ann needs no further introduction; stating her family name would be a redundancy. For those less informed, Dr. Ann is Dr. Ann Wigmore. Dr. Ann was not the only person within the last 100 years to actively promote chlorophyll and wheatgrass for health benefits. Charles Schnabel and later V. Earl Irons made significant strives in promoting wheatgrass/chlorophyll products in America in the early and mid-1900's; however, wheatgrass today is overwhelmingly equated with Ann Wigmore.

By the age of 50, Dr. Ann was battling colon cancer, arthritis, and depression. Like most other 50-year-olds, she also had normal gray hair, a sign of the natural aging process. It was then that she developed her Living Foods Lifestyle® and within several years returned to excellent health. She essentially abandoned her American-style eating habits, to which 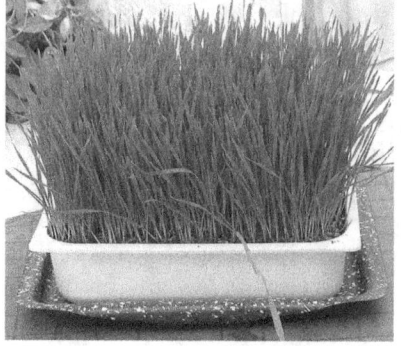 she attributed her deteriorating health. One of the principle aspects of her raw-food lifestyle was adapting the daily habit of drinking fresh liquid chlorophyll. The source of her chlorophyll: fresh wheatgrass juice.

Dr. Ann helped people recover from chronic disorders for 30 years using wheatgrass. She tragically perished in a fire at the age of 83 in 1993. Up until her premature death, she was limber, energetic, and intellectually sharp. Her hair color had even returned to its natural brown.

Indeed, of the many books that she wrote, the one that she is most famous for is *The Wheatgrass Book*.[151] She stated that starting the day with a shot/glass of fresh chlorophyll containing wheatgrass juice is starting the day with a storehouse of vitamins, minerals, hundreds of enzymes, amino acids and oxygen in liquid form.

There are many other benefits of drinking fresh

wheatgrass. The following is a very partial list:[152]

- Normal metabolism causes the constant production of body acids. An excess of acidity in the body weakens bones and teeth, and reduces our immunity from colds and other illnesses. The abundance of alkaline minerals in wheatgrass juice helps to reduce over acidity in the blood.

- Amino acids are the basic structural building units of proteins. Wheatgrass contains 17 amino acids including the eight essentials.

- Speeds up blood circulation and metabolic rate – helping to control weight, thus enhance digestive powers melting the excess fat in the body.

- Protects us from free radicals

- Stimulation and regeneration of the liver

- Destroys harmful germs and microbes

- Contains selenium – (see Chapter 7 – Post Pasteur)

- Requires little energy to digest

- Increases antioxidant levels

- Inhibition of Carcinogens

According to Dr. Theodore M. Rudolph, the daily use of chlorophyll is very beneficial for people suffering from hardening of the arteries (arteriosclerosis). He believes that chlorophyll's ability to combine with oxygen, and its cleansing ability, contributes much to the removal of foreign matter from the walls of the blood vessels.[153]

Grow your own wheatgrass

I was not content to simply stop my poor eating habits that contributed to my heart attack in 2001. The elimination of trans-fats and partially hydrogenated oils undoubtedly slowed down further deterioration of my personal health. I wanted to make a conscious effort to improve my health, and not only maintain the existing status quo.

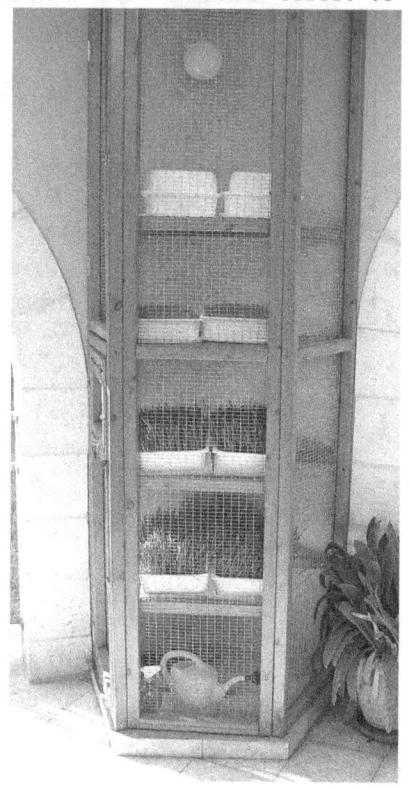

Today I start my day with a shot of wheatgrass, and my purpose for describing here how I grow it is to emphasize that wheatgrass can be grown and enjoyed by anyone; it is not a privilege enjoyed only by the die-hard naturalists and those eating 100% or close to 100% raw and natural food. Growing wheatgrass is something that is doable by anyone. It is also an important step in ingesting a greater percentage of healthy food in our daily diets. While wheatgrass can be (and usually is) grown indoors by many people, I grow it outdoors in an old birdcage that I converted for this endeavor. Interested parties are strongly encouraged to obtain further information from the sources listed at the end of this chapter.

The type of wheatgrass seeds usually used are those

known as 'hard' or 'winter' wheat berries. Like other natural seeds and nuts, their own enzyme inhibitors protect them. This allows them to survive until growing time. Therefore, before planting, the wheatgrass seeds must be sprouted.

Sprouting

The amount of seeds to be prepared depends on the size of the growing trays you will be using. The trays I use are 12½" x 10½" (32cm x 27cm). Fill a wide-mouth jar with one cup of seeds. Secure a piece of nylon screen over the jar and secure it with a rubber band. Rinse the seeds by filling up the jar and spilling out the water several times. Fill the jar with water, and place it in a dark area for approximately 12 hours. After the 12-hour soak, rinse the seeds several times (through the secured nylon screen), and let the jar drain at a 45-degree angle for another 12 hours.

Depending on the season, you may have to modify sprouting procedures; there is no absolute right and wrong. Dr. Ann recommended the 12-hour soak and 12-hour drain time. Dr. Bernard Jensen, well versed in a wide variety of holistic healthcare disciplines, favors planting immediately after the initial 12-hour soak.[154] Steve Meyerowitz, the 'sproutman' and current wheatgrass guru recommends an initial soak of 9-12 hours, rinsing well, then germinating the seeds in a sprouter bag for two days, making sure to rinse at least twice a day.[155] The instruction CD that I received with my wheatgrass juicer recommends soaking for 12 hours and draining for another 12. I seem to obtain best results when soaking for 9 - 12 hours, and draining (with rinsing) for about another 24 hours.

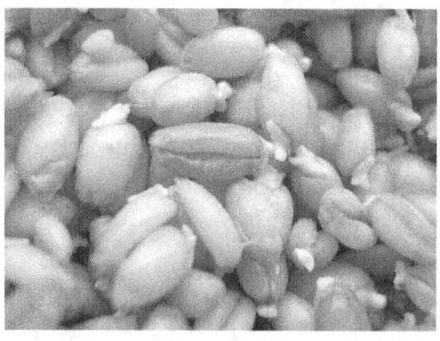 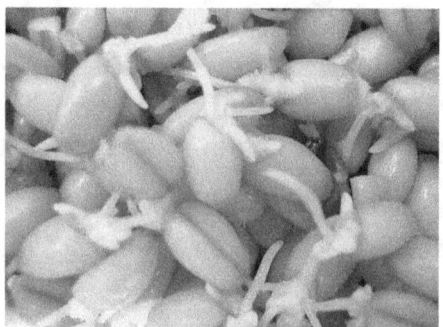

Wheatgrass seeds after 12-hour draining

Wheatgrass seeds after 24-hour draining

Planting

Once sprouted the wheat berries are ready for planting. The seeds are ready to plant when they have doubled in size and the tips of the roots are visible. The tips will be longer if the seeds are drained for 24 and not 12 hours. Fill the tray with an even layer of soil and gently spread the wheat berries over the soil. I favor Dr. Ann's method of not piling up the wheat berry seeds on top of one another. The instruction CD that I mentioned earlier recommends spreading the seeds two or three deep. This is done to promote a thicker harvest. My growing trays have adequate draining holes drilled out of the bottom. Water the seeds (the dirt should be moist and not soaked) and cover the tray with another empty tray

Remove the upper tray when the wheatgrass reaches a height of about one inch and leave in indirect sunlight. Water as necessary in accordance with the weather, humidity and temperature. If the trays are sitting on a flat tray to catch excess water, elevate the upper tray slightly; a couple of pebbles in the corners are adequate. This will allow for all the excess water to drain out of the seeded tray and not be trapped within. The biggest problem I encounter is a greenish blue mold just above soil level, which seems to happen because of over-watering and/or overly hot weather. When the wheatgrass reaches seven to ten inches (18-25 cm) in height, it is ready for harvesting. Use a pair of large scissors to cut it as low as possible.

I cut and juice the wheatgrass first thing in the morning. Once juiced, it should be drunk immediately. Cut wheatgrass can be kept under refrigeration for up to a week. I prepare and plant a new batch every two to two and a half days. You may, if you decide to, harvest your tray a second time. From my experience, this depends on the quality of the first harvest. If it was basically mold free, then I may wait to see how the second batch develops.

Dr. Ann goes into detail on how to recycle the used wheatgrass mats. Here you have a choice on deciding to which doctrine you want to adhere. Dr. Ann's doctrine is organic. She goes with the natural composting to improve and maintain the fertility of soil. For this you must be prepared to wait upwards of three months for this natural process to occur, including the physical place to hold three or so barrels/large trash cans. It helps to obtain earthworms to help 'process' the recycled mats. See references at the end of this chapter.

Changing of the wheatgrass guard

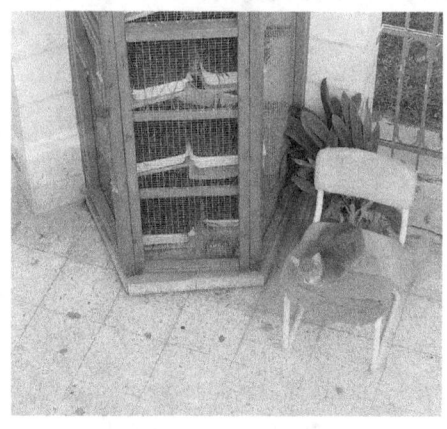

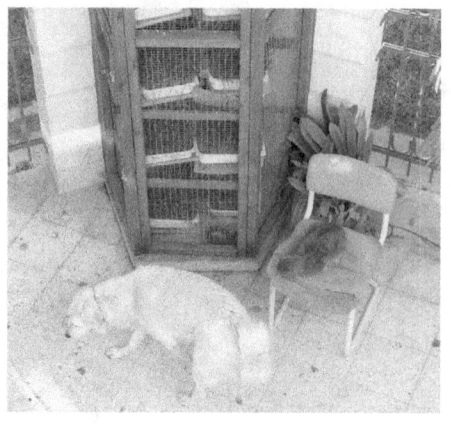

Where's Lambchop? Late as usual!

Nice you decided to show up!

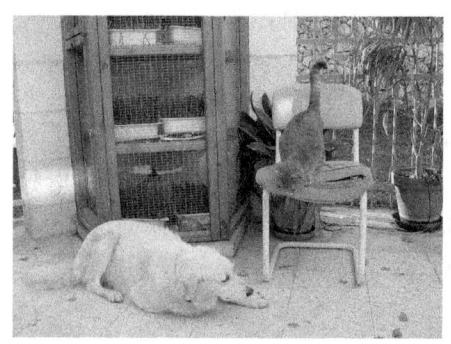

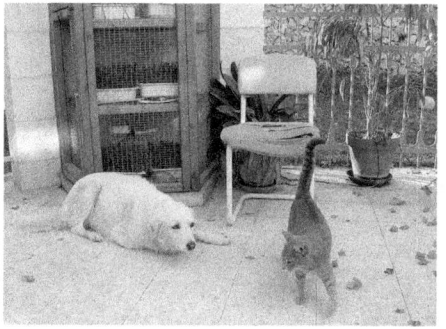

OK, Lambchop, if you're in
place, I'm gonna take off.

Have a nice night off, Gray. See
ya tomorrow, Lambchop.

Another use for wheatgrass seeds

Wheatgrass seeds can also be used to make a healthy, tart and slightly carbonated drink called rejuvelac.[156] After the wheatgrass seeds have sprouted for several days (rinsing twice a day), instead of planting them, place them in a large glass container, and rinse well. Add one quart of water per every cup of wheatgrass seeds, again cover with the nylon screen mesh and let stand for two days (less in summer). When ready, filter through the screen mesh. It should be cloudy, tart but not too sour; if too sour, it may be spoiled. I also pour it through a clean cloth diaper as an additional filtering method. (Diaper? We will encounter diapers again in the next chapter.) Refrigerate and consume within a couple of days.

Return the sprouted seeds back into the large glass container, fill again with water, and the next batch will be ready in another 24 hours. The process can be repeated a third time.

Make very sure that the seeds you are using to make rejuvelac are organic and have not been sprayed with pesticides. Don't forget, the wheatgrass seeds are soaking in what you ultimately will be drinking.

Before filtering the ready rejuvelac, if whitish foam is floating at the top, it can be easily sifted off with a spoon.

I am also a Victoria fan

The name 'Victoria' may not yet be as universal as 'Dr. Ann' so I will present her by her full name, Victoria Boutenko –the same Boutenko mentioned in chapter 4. The Boutenko family arrived to the U.S. from the former Soviet Union. They adapted quite well to American life, which included succumbing to a wide range of 'normal' diseases resulting from eating 'normal' foods. Victoria herself had arrhythmia and edema. She was also obese and depressed. Her husband suffered from painful rheumatoid arthritis and had severe hyperthyroid. Their kids rounded out the list with juvenile diabetes and asthma.

In 1994, the Boutenkos embarked on a diet of entirely raw foods, returned to perfect health, and have since been known as the Raw Family.

Victoria points out in *Green for Life*[157] the anatomical resemblance between chimpanzees and us humans. In fact we both share an approximate 99.4% of the same DNA sequence.[158] There is a good reason for this. Many anthropologists tend to believe that the modern human being evolved from a chimpanzee-like ancestor.[159]

Victoria observed that there is a huge difference in the chimpanzees' eating habits and our own. Chimpanzees do not eat most of the foods that we humans eat. These include all the cooked foods, the starchy carbohydrates, oils and junk food in general. The small amounts of the vegetables we do eat are mostly roots. The chimps on the other hand consume close to 50% of their diet as fruit, and the majority of the remaining 50% as greens.

Modern chimpanzees, however, are not herbivores; they are actually omnivores, like us.[160] Although chimpanzees generally subsist on fruits and greens, they will hunt monkeys on occasion, even when fruits are plentiful.[161] This is not characteristic behavior of a true herbivore.

In direct contrast to the roots (of the greens) that we consume, the chimps eat the leafy part of the vegetable. They eat roots only when there is a shortage of the usual fruits and greens.

The invention of the Victoria Smoothie

Nature has its unique way of protecting its treasures and allowing their survival. The primary structural component of green plants is cellulose. Its strength is what keeps the plant cells rigid and protects the valuable nutrients that are stored inside the cells. For all her motivation and heath awareness, Victoria knew that having to chew the greens to a creamy consistency adequately enough to release the nutrients from their protective cells was not practical for us humans. Enter the high-speed food blender; rupturing the strong cell walls was now accomplished. In addition to the greens, add some fruit into the blender, and the resulting drink is both healthy and tasty.

Blending the greens to a drinkable pulp has advantages over juicing and throwing away the solid byproduct. The cellulose of plants is not digestible by humans. It is an insoluble dietary fiber, in contrast to the soluble fiber which is found in the fruit. Fiber plays an important role in our digestive system. The main purpose of fiber is elimination. If we do not consume enough fiber, the toxic wastes of various sources and dead body cells accumulate in our bodies.

The soluble fiber improves bowel movements by increasing the volume of bulk in the colon. The insoluble fiber acts as a sponge, absorbing toxins. Both types of fiber are necessary for elimination. According to the American Heart Association both types of fiber are associated with a decreased risk of cardiovascular disease.[162]

Varying the greens in our diet also insures the digestion all of the essential amino acids that are vital for protein production.

Introducing the Mike Shlush

What is a Mike Shlush? Basically, it would contain

the same or similar ingredients as a Victoria smoothie. In *Green for Life* Victoria supplies a comprehensive choice of what ingredients and in what amounts to prepare a smoothie. I generally use whatever greens (usually lettuce, coriander, spinach, parsley, etc) that happen to be in the house.

The big difference is in the hardware. Victoria uses a powerful high-speed Vitamix Blender. Its blade spinning at 240 miles per hour will liquefy practically anything she happens to blend; hence the name of her creation – the liquid Victoria smoothie. I am using a 25-year-old Magi mix Food Processor – maybe the only one of its kind still left in the Middle East. The result is not a pure smoothie; it's more like a shlush that still has to be somewhat munched before swallowing – hence the semi-liquid Mike Shlush.

Recommended reading:

The Wheatgrass Book, Ann Wigmore, Avery/Penguin Putnam

Wheatgrass Nature's Finest Medicine, Steve Meyerowitz, Book Publishing Co.

Green For Life, Victoria Boutenko, Raw Family Publishing.

12

Fermenting

Often, the less there is to justify a traditional custom,
the harder it is to get rid of it.
Mark Twain

There are many things that are passed down from
generation to generation. This is known as tradition.
There are things that exist generation after
generation, and eventually peter out. My maternal
grandmother could never understand how it was possible
for me to grow up not learning/knowing Yiddish. My folks
of course understand it, they can still converse in it to some
extent.

My siblings and I are totally Yiddish illiterate. Am I
sorry that as a tot I was not exposed to Yiddish? Of course
I am because during early years, foreign languages seem to
be absorbed easily and naturally. Do I really have the need
for Yiddish in my daily life? Not really, but the idea of
having been able to learn it painlessly and effortlessly
seems to be an unexploited opportunity.

Do I blame my folks for this unutilized opportunity? Not really. I committed a much greater blooper. When Esty and I were married, seven years after my immigration to Israel, my Hebrew was already better than her English. It naturally followed that Hebrew became the daily spoken language in our home.

Nevertheless, I proclaimed that when we will be blessed with children, I would speak with them in English only. With Naamah, the plan got off to a promising start. For the first year of her life, I spoke to her only in English. Then we moved to a different city due to a job change, I started working longer and longer hours, and the rest is well known. I decided to improve this endeavor when Sagi was born, and again when Rakefet was born and of course when Tuval came along.

We have a video movie of baby Tuval correctly answering questions like 'Where is your diaper?' and 'Where is your elbow?' Several years later, diaper and elbow were no longer any part of his vocabulary. That was my blooper, my responsibility. The kids today of course do speak English. This, however, is more to the credit of the school system here and the Simpsons, but they definitely do not speak it with a North American accent.

Tradition is also not necessarily based solely on historical fact. It is also based on how we remember the past, which is not always identical to how the past really was. My folks grew up eating traditionally prepared foods from the traditional kosher kitchen. I have no doubt that in my earliest years this tradition was still in effect. However, like most people, I have very little recollection from those very early years. If you would ask my mom, she would tell you that I was crazy about her lamb chops. The fact that I really don't remember the lamb chops doesn't mean there weren't really lamb chops!

I was born in 1950, but for me, the food tradition at home dates only as far back as I can remember -- 1956? 1960? 1965? And what do I remember about traditional American food as I approached my teen years? It was the hotdogs, hamburgers, fries, pizza, and submarine sandwiches.

Foods known as authentic traditional foods were of course in existence well before the start of my own personal memory or existence. How far back does this tradition go? Not hundreds, but thousands of years. One of the ancient methods of preparing and preserving foods was utilizing natural fermentation. We all know the term fermentation as a process used to produce wine, beer and vinegar. Wine jars dating back more than 7000 years ago have been excavated at Hajji Firuz located in modern day Iran.[163]

In the more general sense, fermentation refers to the conversion of sugar to alcohol using yeast, or the chemical conversion of carbohydrates into alcohols or acids. Fermentation also has some uses exclusive to foods. Fermentation can produce important nutrients which are elements or compounds necessary for contributing to an organism's metabolism, growth, or other functioning. Fermentation also eliminates anti-nutrients (also known as enzyme inhibitors), which are substances that interfere directly with the absorption of vitamins, minerals and other nutrients.

Lacto-fermentation is the process whereby friendly bacteria transform sugars and starches into beneficial lactic acid. Lactic acid acts as a preservative that inhibits pathogenic bacteria (undesirable microorganisms) in the food or drink undergoing fermentation. Recommended sources for additional and technical information regarding fermentation can be found at the website of the Weston A. Price Foundation.

One does not have to be a die-hard naturalist living on a farm somewhere out in the boondocks in order to begin receiving the benefits of fermentation. It is the purpose of this chapter to show you that anyone, in any kitchen, can easily supplement any diet with healthy naturally fermented foods.

Kefir

The culturing of dairy products, found almost universally among pre-industrialized peoples, enhanced the enzyme content of those products. Kefir is a drink prepared by inoculating milk with the grains of previous kefir batches. Kefir grains are a combination of bacteria and yeasts in a matrix of proteins, lipids and sugars. They contain over 30 probiotic bacteria proven highly beneficial to humans. The term probiotic refers to live microorganisms which when administered in adequate amounts, confer a health benefit on the host.[164]

As the term itself implies, probiotic is the opposite of antibiotic. Probiotic: 'pro' refers to 'for'; 'biotic' refers to 'life' -- the result, 'life promoting'. Antibiotic: 'anti' refers to 'against'; 'biotic' refers to 'life' -- the result, 'against life'. The protein contained in cultured (lacto-fermented) dairy products is the very highest quality available for human consumption. And as a bonus for those still worried about their cholesterol levels, an anti-cholesteremic milk factor (lowering of blood levels of cholesterol) has been discovered in fermented milk and fermented milk products.[165]

Homemade kefir is very easy to make. You do need to start with a small handful of kefir grains. The Internet provides a good source for finding kefir grains; there are a number of worldwide forums dedicated to kefir, kefir making and how and where to obtain grains. I prepare kefir using a small wide-mouth Mason jar. Simply put the kefir grains in the jar, add a glass of milk, and gently stir or agitate. The jar should not be more than 2/3 full. Initially, the fresh milk will thicken until it obtains a consistency much like smooth yogurt. With longer fermentation, it separates into a layer of thick curd floating on top of greenish whey. The mixture should be shaken or stirred two or three times per day.

I like the Mason jars because they can be closed hermetically for shaking/agitating without having the mixture splash out. Esty is still very unused to sharing the kitchen with me -- even when I don't mess up! I usually leave the lid on the Mason jar loose enough to allow carbon dioxide produced in the fermentation process to escape from the jar. Leaving the jar closed tightly will give the kefir more of a sour taste.

Fermentation is dependent on temperature, time and the activity of the specific grains. The longer it ferments, the tarter the taste. As a general guide kefir will ferment twice as fast at 86°F (30°C) as at 68°F (20°C), but remember, as you approach 100°F (37°C) degrees, the grains lose their potency. Fermentation time takes between 24 to 48 hours. Once the kefir has cultured to your liking, strain it through a sieve using a spoon to gently separate the kefir drink from the grains. If you prefer to drink it cold, refrigerate as necessary before drinking. Return the Kefir grains into the Mason jar with fresh milk and repeat the process.

Most any type of milk can be used -- even dead pasteurized homogenized cow milk. At the end of chapter 7 (Post-Pasteur), I did mention without going into any detail the existence of pro and con camps regarding homogenization and heart disease.[166]

The ultimate solution -- use goat's milk! First, if you are not sure where you stand on the homogenization issue, there is no need to homogenize goat's milk. Fat molecules of goat's milk are one-fifth the size of cow's milk.[167] You can verify this yourself. The next time you are in the dairy section of your local supermarket, check out the commercially sold goat's milk. It is pasteurized; however, it is not homogenized.

There are a number of health advantages to using goat's milk, especially raw (unpasteurized) goat's milk.

- Goats are among the healthiest and hardiest of domestic animals.[168] They are naturally immune to diseases, such as tuberculosis.[169]

- Goats are clean by nature.[170] Cows are not. A cow's 'personal hygiene would embarrass a pig'.[171]

- The molecules of goat's milk are closer in size and composition to human milk, making it easier to digest. Goat's milk protein is also substantially less allergenic than cow's milk protein in susceptible individuals.[172]

- Our bodies can digest goat's milk in about 20 minutes; it takes two to three hours to digest cow's milk.[173]

- Goat's milk contains a unique essential balance of vitamins, minerals, proteins, carbohydrates, enzymes and fats; it is one of the few whole foods that are able to sustain life.[174]

- Goat's milk is the highest source of selenium (Chapter 7) of any of the milks.[175]

- Fresh goat's milk (like mother's milk) is alkaline and has a tendency to neutralize acids in the body.[176] Cow's milk has an acid reaction.[177]

- Goat's milk differs from cow's milk in that it contains more of the essential fatty acids (linoleic and arachidonic) and it has a greater percentage of medium and short-chain saturated fatty acids. These differences suggest that the fat of goat's milk may be more readily digested than that of cow's milk.[178]

- Crohn's disease is caused by the microorganism Mycobaterium avium subspecies paratuberculosis, or MAP which is common in U.S. dairy herds. The MAP in cow's milk fails to be killed by conventional pasteurization. Transmission of MAP is passed from infected cattle to humans through cow's milk. No disease like MAP affects goats.[179]

- A controversial drug called rBGH (Recombinant Bovine Growth Hormone) is used quite extensively by most dairies in the U.S. It causes cows to produce more milk. rBGH is a product of genetic engineering. A higher rate of cattle disease is reported among cattle being given rBHG which results in a greater use of antibiotics. These antibiotics are passed down to the milk.[180]   Incidentally, rBGH use was approved by the FDA in 1993.

♥ ♥ ♥

The milk I use (when I can obtain it) is fresh raw goat's (or sheep's) milk. I will have to clarify somewhat what I mean by fresh. Raw milk of any type, as in many states in the U.S.A., is not marketed over the counter for human consumption. Finding sources is by word of mouth, friend brings friend. The problem is that my present source is a couple of hours drive away. It is also not available all year around -- depending on the parturition season. This means that most of the milk that I buy at one time winds up in the freezer, so technically it's not really fresh by the time I use it. After thawing out though, it still makes great kefir.

Over time, the Mason jar becomes 'not very aesthetic'. I have a couple of spare Mason jars on hand so that when one enters the dishwasher, there is a spare ready. Make very sure that the kefir is not exposed to chlorinated water! This means that all jars, utensils etc. must be bone dry before using them. There are those who will use only non-chlorinated water for cleaning all utensils being exposure to kefir. Following are other tips for taking care of your kefir grains:

Severe cold (freezing temperatures) or heat (over 100°F/40°C) can damage the grains. Last summer's heat almost killed off my grains altogether. I do not believe that summer daytime temperatures in my kitchen went over 100°F, however, the grains stopped growing, and they shrank down in size. Keeping the kefir in the fridge during the hottest part of the day seemed to help the grains to recuperate. Another option – during the cooler winter months, the grains grow and multiply rapidly. I accumulate the excessive grains and refrigerate them in a 'milk bath' and use them to reinforce the kefir grains in the hot summer months. Every couple of weeks I replace the milk.

I do not let the grains come in contact with metal, although there are those who claim this is not important. The spoon I use to separate the grains from the kefir is actually a plastic won-ton soup spoon. The mesh of the strainer sieve is plastic/nylon. Do not keep your kefir/grains in direct sunlight. When stirring or filtering the grains, do not squeeze them. Be gentle!

Keep in mind that the grains are living entities. As you would not want to do without food, neither would they. The only exception to this if you need to store the grains. There are proper methods for dehydrating them and preparation for freezing. Check out the forums or other relevant articles on the net.

The living grains are constantly growing, which allows one to share them with friends every couple of weeks. If it isn't already obvious, the grains are also edible.

Fresh Cream Cheese

Usually one of the first things I do after obtaining fresh raw goat's or sheep's milk directly from the farm is to use the first couple of liters to make a couple of small tubs of cream cheese (14-17.5 oz / 400-500 grams).

When I first started making my own cream cheese, I followed standard popular recipes which involved slowly heating the fresh milk to 180°F (82°C), and then adding vinegar or lemon juice. This caused the milk to curdle and separate from the liquid whey; the cheese curds were then separated from the whey by straining. While this did supply me with homemade cheese and homemade whey, I did realize eventually that this was partially self-defeating.

Although I did produce a product without any artificial preservatives, the heating was still killing off the beneficial enzymes in the process, so what was I ultimately gaining?

My present method of making cream cheese is based on a simple recipe by the Weston A. Price Foundation head Ms. Sally Fallon Morell.[181] Raw milk, with all of its natural enzymes intact, separates into milk curds and whey when left unrefrigerated for several days (longer in winter, shorter in summer – it's a function of temperature).

Cheese making – summer months

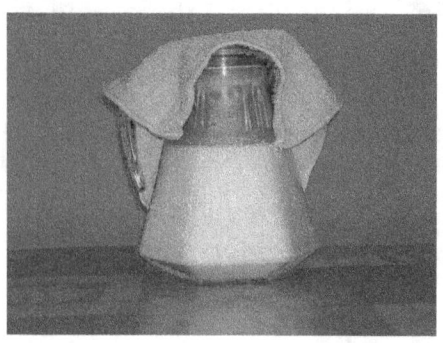 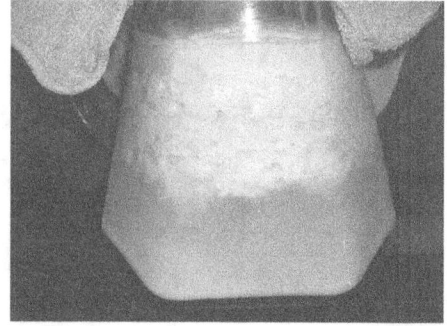

Day 1: Pour raw milk into a large glass container.

Within a day or two (or three, depending upon the temperature), the whey separates from the cheese curds.

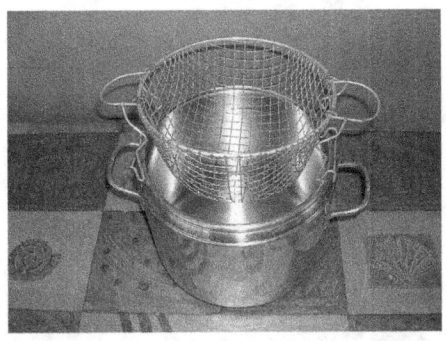

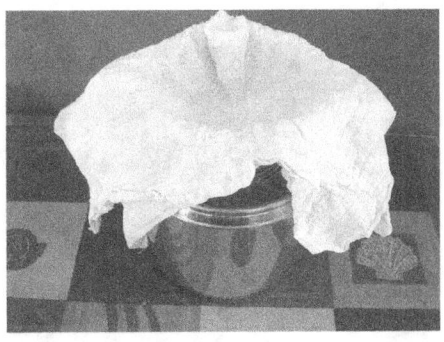

Prepare a large pot (stainless steel). On top of it, place a drain screen (same as used for draining the oil from deep frying).

Place a cloth diaper (or cheese cloth) into the strainer.

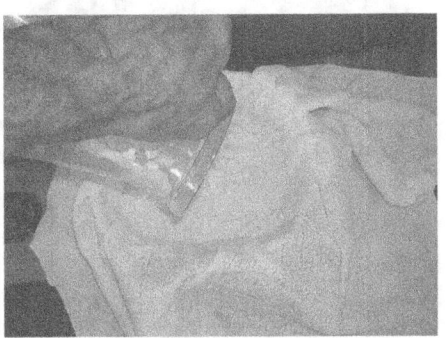

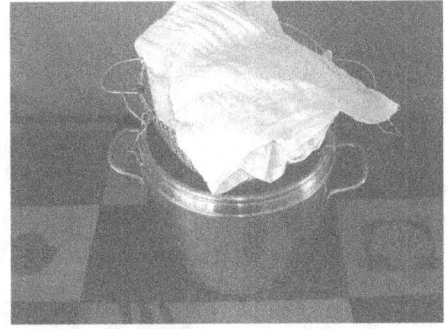

Empty the contents of the container (whey and cheese curds).

Drain, and place as is in refrigerator for several more hours.

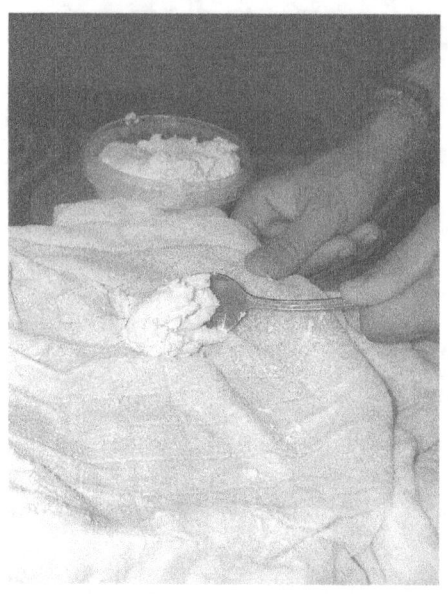

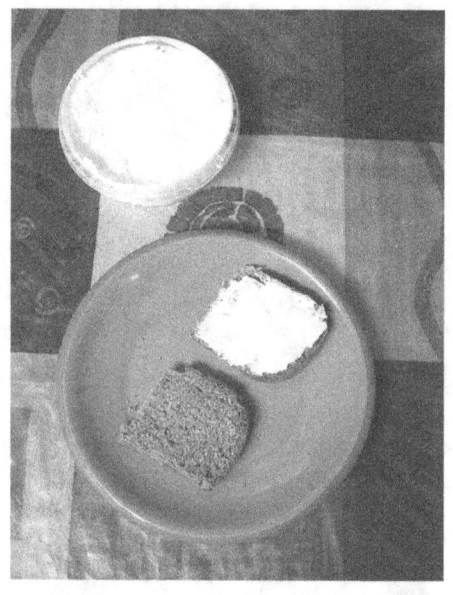

Store the cheese in containers -- use a spoon to scrape off the diaper.

With some fresh homemade whole wheat bread straight out of the oven – Bon Appetit!

I learned at the beginning of last winter that leaving milk out in a cold kitchen is basically leaving it in a 'not very cold refrigerator'. It simply doesn't want to separate! I found a novel way to speed up the separation. Use a simple yogurt maker; the heat is very mild. If you remember the test for enzyme tolerance from Chapter 4, the heated yogurt maker does not approach being uncomfortable when handling. It does not damage the enzymes and separates the milk within two days. The major difference is using a number of regular-sized glasses that fit into the yogurt maker instead of one single large vessel to house the milk while waiting for it to separate into curds and whey.

Cheese making – winter months

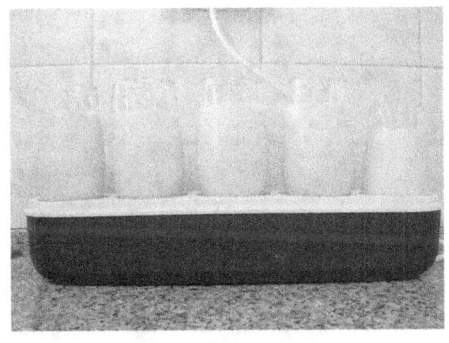

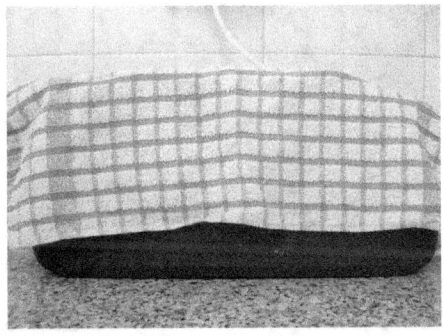

Day 1: Pour raw milk into separate glasses and put in low heat yogurt maker.

Cover glasses completely to keep them heated evenly.

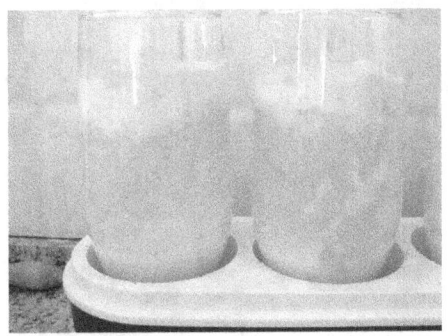

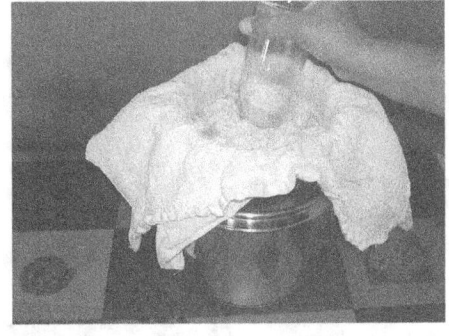

Within a day or two (or three, depending upon the temperature), the whey separates from the cheese curds.

Pour into diaper-lined strainer and continue as above.

Making the cheese dryer

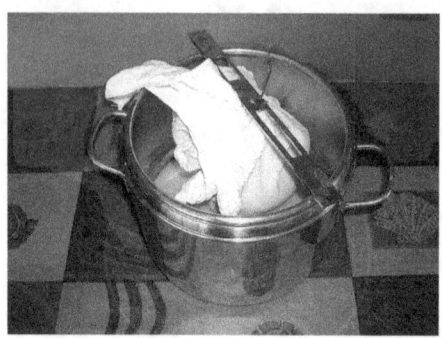

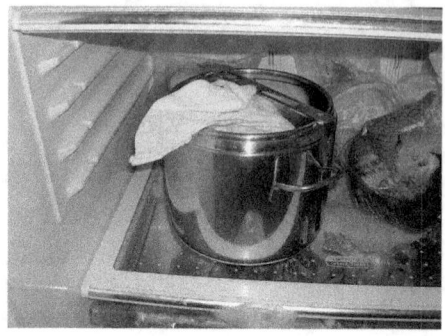

After initial draining, tie the diaper/cheese cloth into a bundle and suspend it so it does not touch the whey.

Place as is into the refrigerator for another eight hours.

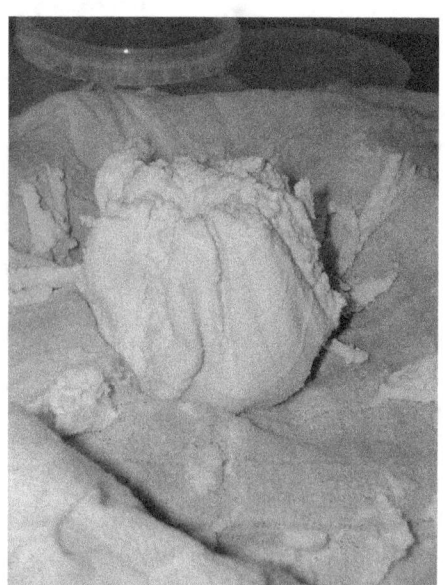

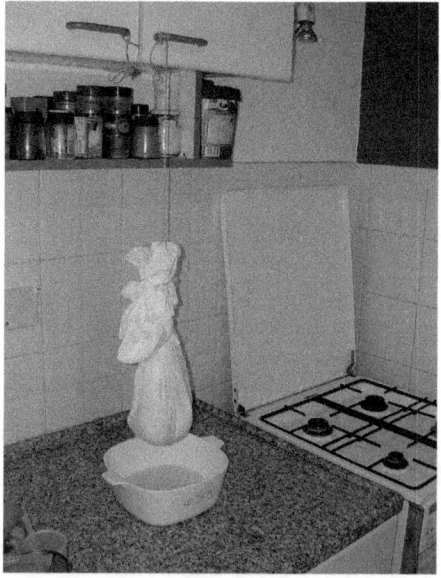

Voila! Open the diaper. The cheese is less creamy and more solid.

This is another way to hang the cheese to dry, however, not especially recommended if your wife has things to do in the kitchen…......

Whey

Does it seem strange that I make my own cheese? After all, I can, and usually do bring back some homemade goat's cheese from my milk supplier. The reason why I make my own cream cheese is because I am not only interested in the cheese itself, but interested in the byproduct that is produced in the process.

I am referring to the yellowish colored liquid that separates from the cheese known as 'whey'. Whey is an excellent source of protein, vitamins, minerals and lactose. Historically, the cheese industry viewed whey as the waste material in cheese production and either discarded it or used it as a fertilizer. Recently, its worth as both an animal feed and a food ingredient has been recognized. Its price has soared to about 79 cents a pound[182] -- a good cash item for cheese diaries. The founding fathers of medicine, Hippocrates, and later Galen, recommended whey to their patients to cure a variety of diseases.[183]

It is also indispensable for making homemade fermented vegetables, grains and beverages. Whey is rich in lactic acid, which speeds up the process of fermentation. It was through this process of lacto-fermentation that our forefathers were able to preserve vegetables before the invention of freezers and canning methods.[184]

My first homemade fermented dish made with whey was sauerkraut. The recipe and directions come from, where else, again Ms. Sally Fallon Morell.[185] Even a lifelong non-kitchen person such as me can follow her easy to understand recipes.

How do I discard excess whey that I have no foreseeable use for? I pour it over the recycled soil mats before replanting new wheatgrass seeds. It may not have the same effect as using Dr. Maynard Murray's method of using diluted ocean water for its rich balanced mineral content as a natural fertilizer;[186] however, it is a way of natural recycling.

13

Aw Nuts……..

You are as old as your arteries.
Hanna Kroeger[187]

There are a number of expressions that one uses to express great dissatisfaction at any given moment, such as 'oh sh--' and other four-letter words. People who are more cultured and who do not want to swear in public but still need to verbalize current dismay can safely say 'Aw nuts!' instead, and still retain their civilized identities.

Another usage of nuts: Esty at times (if not most of the time) thinks that I'm nuts. And this was even before some of the eating habits I have acquired since my heart attack, which she still has trouble adjusting to. But I have a license to be nuts. James Bond, 007, has a license to kill. I survived my heart attack. I later survived the statins; I earned the license to be nuts.

Seriously though, what made me start adding various types of nuts to my diet? It came about with my changing lifestyle, specifically leaving my last job and starting a job involving shift work. Basically I was interested in increasing my knowledge regarding health pitfalls to watch out for now that I was leaving the normal day/night schedule. There was a necessity to alter my sleep habits according to my new work schedule. This involved both the afternoon/evening shift (arriving home after one a.m.) and later, the graveyard shift -- starting either ten or eleven p.m. and arriving home in the morning when most people have already had breakfast and on their way to work.

Published information was not especially encouraging:

- *Heart problems also have been noted more often among shift workers than day workers.....Researchers found that the longer people worked shifts, the more likely they were to develop heart disease....*[188]

- *These results suggest that shiftwork has direct and unfavourable effects on cardiac autonomic activity and that this might be one mechanism via which shiftwork increases the risk of cardiovascular disease. It is postulated that sleep loss could be one mediator of the association between shiftwork and cardiovascular health.*[189]

What are the possible consequences of altering my natural circadian rhythm, and what can I do to minimize the resulting health hazards?

Circadian rhythms are important in determining our sleeping and feeding patterns. There are clear patterns within our 24-hour normal day/night schedule of hormone production, brain wave activity, cell regeneration and other biological functions. Anyone who has ever experienced jetlag knows firsthand what happens when his/her circadian rhythms are interfered with. Common symptoms are fatigue during the daytime, disorientation and insomnia at nighttime and possible mood disorders. This circadian clock is normally timed to the Earth's natural light and dark cycles, which is perfect for the regular daytime job.

Most circadian rhythms are controlled by the SupraChiasmatic Nucleus or SCN, which acts as the body's clock. The SCN rests in a part of the brain just above the point where the optic nerves cross. Light that reaches photoreceptors in the eye retina creates signals that travel along the optic nerve to the SCN. Signals from the SCN travel to several brain regions, including the pineal gland. This gland responds to light-induced signals by switching off production of the hormone melatonin.

For people maintaining the normal day/night schedule, melatonin level rises during nighttime sleep. It reaches a peak between eleven p.m. and two a.m., and then drops significantly during sunrise. One of the major problems of working shift work is not getting enough high-quality sleep. This in turn results in a vicious cycle of sorts; the lack of nighttime sleep causes a reduction in melatonin production and the shortage of adequate levels of melatonin prevent us from getting enough sleep! Adequate melatonin levels are also associated with assisting us in dealing with stress, and lowering blood pressure and the risk of heart rhythm problems.[190]

An interesting study involving the seeds of plants may shed some light on the importance of melatonin to cardio health in us Homo sapiens:

This level of melatonin is much higher than the known physiological concentrations in the blood of many vertebrates. Since the seed, particularly its germ tissue, is highly vulnerable to oxidative stress and damage, we surmise that melatonin, a free radical scavenger, might be present as an important component of its antioxidant defense system.[191]

How then is it possible to raise melatonin levels, besides trying to simulate night conditions during the daytime by sleeping in a totally dark room or at least covering the eyes? The answer is via our diet. More specifically, a handful of nuts helps raise our melatonin level, which ultimately helps us sleep better. Nuts contain important nutrients and beneficial phytonutrients and also have many characteristics vital for keeping our cardio systems running smoothly.

Walnuts contain melatonin and also contribute to the antioxidative capacity of the blood.[192] Walnuts are relatively high in arginine, an essential amino acid. Essential amino acids cannot be synthesized by the organism and therefore must be obtained via food diet. Amino acids function as building blocks in protein biosynthesis. In the body, arginine is converted into nitric oxide (NO), a chemical that helps keep the inner walls of blood vessels smooth and allows blood vessels to relax. Both atherosclerosis and acute coronary events increase when NO levels decline.[193] Foods high in arginine help the body produce its own nitric oxide.

Almonds are an excellent source of the amino acid tryptophan. Tryptophan is a precursor (forerunner or predecessor) of melatonin. The building blocks for natural melatonin production in the body include sufficient amounts of vitamin B6, vitamin B3 and most importantly, tryptophan.

In SASHA I discussed the serious consequences of reduced levels of brain serotonin levels resulting from the use of statins. Tryptophan is also a precursor for serotonin, which is an additional reason to eat almonds. Serotonin is the neuro-transmitter responsible for feelings of well-being, mood, self-confidence and concentration. The only source for serotonin in the brain is tryptophan. It cannot be converted from any other substance. Some serotonin is converted in the pineal gland to melatonin. Melatonin production is inversely proportional to that of serotonin, a chemical.[194] Generally during the night, when the mind is less active, less serotonin and more melatonin is produced.

Almonds contain much more vitamin E than all other nuts, and most other foods in general.[195] Vitamin E, a fat-soluble vitamin, is an antioxidant vitamin involved in the metabolism of all cells. It protects essential fatty acids from oxidation in the body cells, helps deactivate free radicals and prevents breakdown of body tissues. Almond skins contain flavonoids which act synergistically (combined effect greater than separate individual effects) with vitamins C and E to enhance LDL resistance to oxidation.[196] Hanna Kroeger, a staunch advocate of natural healing methods recommends an almond drink spanning the course of 30 days to be done once a year.[197]

Peanut lovers (peanuts are technically legumes, and not nuts) will be happy to hear that they contain significant amounts of both tryptophan and arginine.

Do nuts have a downside? They may if proper precautions are not taken. First of all, nuts, like grains, contain numerous enzyme inhibitors that can put a real strain on the digestive mechanism if consumed in excess. In SASHA I mentioned that I soaked my homemade granola (incidentally oats are also a good source of tryptophan) to neutralize the phytates (enzyme inhibitors).[198] Nuts are easier to digest and their nutrients are more readily available if they are first soaked[199] in water and then dried. Besides neutralizing the enzyme inhibitors, this can increase the vitamin and mineral content. Before the food revolution of the last century, traditional people always soaked or partially sprouted their seeds and nuts before they were eaten. You can of course make the nuts crunchy again by roasting; however, extended roasting at high temperature kills the enzymes and damages the nuts' delicate fats.

Is there a downside to peanuts? First of all, peanuts contain an especially high amount of enzyme inhibitors. They must never be eaten raw. Secondly, a study performed in 1988 showed peanut oil to be unexpectedly atherogenic for monkeys, rabbits, and rats.[200]

Keep in mind that walnuts, as opposed to many other types of nuts, are extremely susceptible to rancidity.[201] In warm conditions they quickly go rancid particularly after shelling. Heat, light and humidity will speed spoilage. The best way to preserve them is to buy them in the shell, or keep them in an airtight container in the refrigerator or even in the freezer.

Neutralizing the enzyme inhibitors in nuts is not enough. It is important to understand the connection between nuts and Essential Fatty Acids omega-3 and omega-6 -- and the infamous O6/O3 ratio (chapter 9). I will discuss this further in Chapter 18.

14

The Next 20,000

*Life is like riding a bicycle. To keep your
balance you must keep moving.*
Albert Einstein

The next 20,000? The next 20,000 what? 20,000
Leagues Under the Sea?* I mentioned in the preface
that anyone who has read SASHA would probably
be able to guess what the 20,000 stands for; and indeed it is
the next 20,000 kilometers (12,427 miles) of bicycle riding.
It will be a bit difficult to explain this significance in only a
paragraph or two; it relates to my post heart attack period
when the side effects of the statins I was prescribed started
taking their toll.

The effects totally disrupted my profession and
personal life. What had started as being simply a tool to
maintain physical conditioning in post heart attack life, the
bike riding slowly became a total obsession. It was how I

---

* Sorry Jules

started my day every morning; it was the only thing I enjoyed doing during the day. The daily riding improved my stamina, which allowed me to take very long bike rides over the weekend. After a few months of riding, I set my annual goal to 4,000 kilometers (2,485mi) which was eventually revised to 5,000 kilometers (3,107mi), and finally to 5,215 (an exact 100 kilometers a week average for the entire year).

In fact, an entire chapter in SASHA was devoted to my personal race to get to that 5,215th kilometer by year's end. Does this obsession sound a little strange? It should; welcome to the world of statin side effects. That is basically what prompted me to write SASHA in the first place.

At the end of that first riding year, I picked my goal for the new riding year based upon my improved stamina over the previous couple of months. The new goal: a 140km (87-mile) average per week for the entire year. This is basically how SASHA ended, reaching the 12,570km (7,810mi) goal by the end that second riding year. The goal I set for myself for the third riding year was to reach a cumulative total of 20,000km (12,427mi). A goal is a goal is a goal. Towards the end of that third year I was averaging 180km (112mi) per week for the last month and a half in order to obtain this goal. And I did reach it.

I mentioned earlier that one of the benefits of writing a book is the personal research one does when working on the project. Yes, writing a book like this is definitely a project. I discovered when writing SASHA that sometimes a single article or even a single sentence is enough to kindle an urge to dig up more information regarding a new idea.

Grisanti? Who is Dr. Grisanti?

Dr. Ronald Grisanti authors one of the newsletters I subscribe to. Why is Dr. Grisanti an authority to me? Basically, I share his views on the real causes of heart disease. He is not a believer in the conventional lipid hypothesis. I share his visions of the non-role of cholesterol and saturated fat with regards to the real cause of heart disease.

One newsletter was headlined with 'Do you want to prevent having a heart attack?' That certainly is a headline that talks my language. After all, I did have one. The gist of the newsletter was that long-duration, low-intensity aerobics do not offer us protection against suddenly experiencing a fatal heart attack; in fact they 'can actually speed up your trip to the grave' as he put it.

That particular line rang a bell for me as I was reading it. Then it rang a gong!

The Bell

What was it that rang the bell? Dr. Grisanti mentioned that Jim Fixx, author of *Complete Book of Running*, had a fatal heart attack… while running.

The Gong

Dr. Grisanti specifically mentioned marathon runners as common fatal heart attack victims. It is said that a picture is worth a thousand words. In this case, I think that this direct quote from SASHA will drive the point home.

Do I plan to continue bike riding?

Definitely! And while on the subject of bike riding and physical exercise in general, I would like to point out that exercising alone does not provide any guarantee against heart attacks and/or an even worse scenario - not surviving a heart attack.

A recent event provided good proof of that. Brian Maxwell, the creator of Power Bars (convenient energy bars used by athletes to give them an energy boost while competing), died this week (April 2004) of a heart attack at the age of 51. What is significant here is that he was a former world-class marathon runner. In 1977, Maxwell was ranked as the third best marathon runner in the world by Track and Field News.

While on the subject of runners, it was 20 years ago (1984) that Jim Fixx had a massive heart attack while jogging and died immediately. He was 52 at the time. It was Fixx's best-selling book "Complete Book of Running" that started the big jogging craze in the seventies.[202]

Was I partially barking up the wrong tree? It was my intention at the time that Fixx's great personal endurance was not enough to keep him healthy. The implication was that if his eating habits were poor then even his fantastic fitness would not guarantee his good health. I am not personally familiar with Maxwell's specific 'Power Bars'. I do know, however, that many health stores sell convenient power/energy bar type snacks for athletes that contain partially hydrogenated fat. I repeat, partially hydrogenated fat ingredients being sold by 'health stores'!

Dr. Grisanti likens the effects of long-duration, low-intensity aerobics on the heart to an old VW Beetle engine. The VW engine, small and economical, runs all day on a single tank of gas. What happens if that same VW with the small economic engine with four full-sized adults sitting in it suddenly has to go up a big hill full speed and needs the power of a Ferrari? Simply put, it cannot handle the load.

How many times have you heard about someone having a heart attack after lifting something heavy, or suddenly after receiving very bad news? Sound familiar? Not being able to temporarily handle the sudden load?

Dr. Grisanti promotes the use of high-intensity 'Grizzly Bear Intervals' several times a week instead of the basic daily aerobic exercising that is prevalent today.[203] Why the name Grizzly Bear? It is based on the simple principle that during aerobic exercise sessions, one should do several sets of exercise at a pace as if a hungry grizzly bear was chasing you. Dr. Grisanti himself states that he didn't invent Grizzly Bear Interval training. However, he has fine-tuned it into a very precise way of exercising.

A check through the medical literature shows that this trend of thought is by no means a new idea. There have been quite of few studies conducted on this subject through the years.

As early as 1990 a study was done on subjects that had already undergone coronary bypass surgery. It concluded that interval type exercise was preferable over constant exercise:

Exercise training according to the I (exertion and recovery phases alternate each minute) method involves both the aerobic and anaerobic capacity of the organism, whereas exercise training according to the C method (constant exertion) involves only oxidative capacity. After coronary bypass surgery, the I method is better suited to increase physical performance and is more effective in economizing the cardiac function.[204]

This particular study mentioned both aerobic and anaerobic capacities. A person utilizes his/her muscles to perform physical work. This is accomplished through muscle contraction. Contraction can be performed only when biochemical energy is converted into mechanical energy. Two types of biochemical energy are involved.

- Aerobic: energy is supplied to the muscles in the presence of oxygen.

- Anaerobic: energy is supplied to the muscles in the absence of oxygen

Aerobic activities are typically of a low to moderate-intensity and can be continued over a considerable amount of time. Walking and jogging would be examples of aerobic activities. Anaerobic activities are very intense and for that reason can only be continued for a very limited time. Running a 100-meter sprint at full speed would be an example of an anaerobic activity. While aerobic fitness is a characteristic of the person as a whole, anaerobic fitness is a local characteristic of the muscle or local muscle group because of its independence on blood and oxygen supply to the area.

A popular worldwide test for measuring anaerobic fitness is the Wingate Anaerobic Test (WAnT). It was developed at the Department of Research and Sport Medicine of the Wingate Institute for Physical Education and Sport in Israel in the seventies.

> *It is used as a standard in accessing muscle power, muscle endurance and fatigability. It has also been used as a reproducible, standardized task that can help analyze physiologic and cognitive responses to supramaximal exercise.*[205]

In 1998 a study showed that skeletal muscle fatigue develops in both high-intensity and also low-intensity exercise; however, it was demonstrated that these are two totally separate fatigue mechanisms. What is interesting is that the low-intensity exercises caused the same pathological intracellular chemical imbalances that are found in heart failure patients.

> *We conclude that with high-intensity exercise perturbations of $Na+$ and $K+$ in muscle cells may contribute to fatigue, whereas with endurance type of exercise and in heart failure patients the skeletal muscle fatigue is more likely to reside in the intracellular control of $Ca2+$ release and reuptake.* [206]

Basically, there has been a substantial amount of research done proving the advantages of short duration high-intensity exercise, over long-duration low-intensity workouts – a few more examples:

- *There is an inverse association between relative intensity of physical activity (an individual's perceived level of exertion) and risk of CHD, even among men not satisfying current activity recommendations.*[207]

- *It was concluded that relatively brief but intense sprint training can result in an increase in both glycolytic and oxidative enzyme activity, maximum short-term power output, and VO2 max.*[208]

- *We conclude that short sprint interval training (approximately 15 min of intense exercise over 2 wk) increased muscle oxidative potential and doubled endurance capacity during intense aerobic cycling in recreationally active individuals.*[209]

- *High-intensity aerobic interval exercise is superior to moderate exercise for increasing VO2peak (peak oxygen uptake) in stable CAD-patients. As VO2peak seems to reflect a continuum between health and cardiovascular disease and death, the present data may be useful in designing effective training programmes for improved health in the future.*[210]

- *These results indicate that high-intensity cycling training in 14 sessions improves enzyme activities of anaerobic and aerobic metabolism.*[211]

And finally, the importance of adequate rest periods and *not* working out every day:

However, performance did not improve in a short training programme that did not include days for recovery, which suggests that muscle fibres suffer fatigue or injury.[212]

The fact that I am learning about this now when the facts have been known for quite some time is actually not surprising. I wonder how many people in the Western world suffering from heart disease have ever heard of Dr. Uffe Ravnskov. It is the Western world that is suffering from heart disease today. He is undoubtedly the spiritual father of the ANTI 'saturated fat and cholesterol cause heart disease' movement that is today gaining momentum. The first edition of Dr. Ravnskov's classic book *The Cholesterol Myths* was first published 16 years ago. How many new cases of heart disease cropped up in the last 16 years during the present reigning lipid hypothesis era?

In SASHA, I went into detail regarding the accepted way and widely publicized method of calculating resting and maximum heart rate for exercise workouts. The maximum rate calculations given were based on starting with a pulse calculation of 220, and subtracting various amounts according to variables of the exerciser (age, etc).

Actually, this widely published formula for maximum heart rate has no scientific merit for use in exercise physiology and related fields.[213] Dr. Grisanti also claims that this calculation will be missing the boat for most people. It will be adequate for about one third of the people using it, but the calculations will be high for one third of others, and low for the other third.

Dr. Grisanti calculates what resting, basic training level and maximum aerobic heart rate should be; however, his calculations are entirely different, and not based upon the 220 starting point.

He instructs the exerciser to perform an exact number of sets tailored personally for anyone using them, which takes into consideration the present fitness of the exerciser. This allows the exerciser to stop the daily exercise before entering the over-training stage, which is counterproductive to maintaining good health. Dr. Grisanti puts a great deal of emphasis on making sure not to over exercise. There are inherent dangers in strenuous exercise, which can, and do, result in the death of supposedly very fit people who are in excellent health.[214]

He recommends walking, stationary bike riding or similar methods as the best way to implement the Grizzly Bear Interval workout. These types of exercise lend themselves well to the accurate adherence to exercising according to the calculated pulse rates.

What attracts me to Grisanti's approach to exercising is that I am an analytic type of person. I often go by numbers when doing something. In SASHA, I had the goal to reach 5,000km, and then revised it to exceed 5215. The next year I chose the 140km weekly average for the year. Numbers are something that can be measured. If they are in any way related to a personal goal to obtain something, it makes the whole mission measurable and accountable.

That said, I personally do not like stationary bikes. I like the real bike, fresh air, sunshine, even if the sunshine is in the middle of the hot summer, or the fresh air is in the middle of the cold winter. I simply enjoy the outside bike riding.

Fresh air vs. inside air -- is there really a difference? The home/apartment/office is a source of a myriad of dangerous materials that influence the air quality.[215] The list includes, but is not limited to: combustion sources such as oil, gas, kerosene, coal, wood, and tobacco products; building materials; asbestos-containing insulation; wet or damp carpet; formaldehyde from cabinetry or furniture made of certain pressed wood products; products for household cleaning and maintenance; products for personal care, or hobbies; central heating and cooling systems and humidification devices; air fresheners; the use of solvents in cleaning and hobby activities; cleaning products and pesticides in housekeeping, etc. High-pollutant concentrations can remain in the air for long periods after some of these activities.

The question is: Is my bike riding more like long-duration aerobatic stationary bike riding, or closer to the Grizzly Bear Interval workout? It's probably a combination of both. After reading about his calculations, I did my next ride in the neighborhood with a pulse meter in order to get the feel of where my resting, maximum and duration laps are according to his calculations. Does this mean that every time I take a ride I am always monitoring my pulse? The answer is no. However, it has changed my awareness of how I ride if it is for exercise purposes only.

I choose my daily route according to how I want to exercise for the day. I now separate my easy bike stroll days from days when I go for the grizzly bear style workout. It is also a good solution for those days when I happen to be in a big hurry and want to finish a good workout in a minimum amount of time.

Grizzly bear intervals comprise only the first half of Dr. Grisanti's exercise workout. The second part involves strength training and its importance to overall muscle tone. Dr. Grisanti advocates the Grunt and Growl Strength Training method, in which the exerciser reaches his own personal momentary muscular failure point following only one set of each specific exercise at a predetermined weight/resistance. Similar to his grizzly bear workouts, Dr. Grisanti spells out a very detailed way of working out in the gym. This includes how the exerciser can determine his/her own exercise workout weights to be used.

Another source of information, one that I consider to be most reliable and informative, also advocates working out in a gym in addition to doing some type of aerobatic workouts. The source: Mr. Anthony Colpo.

Who is Anthony Colpo?

Anthony Colpo is not a university professor, nor associate professor. He is not a medical doctor; he is not a doctor of any sort. He is a certified fitness professional. I guess in my college days we would have called him a physical trainer or 'jock' for short. I don't know if the term is still used today, but you remember the jock stereotype: a 250lb illiterate running back that runs the 100 meters in 11 seconds; or the scholarship to the 6'6" guard that hits 70% of his three pointers. Not only that, but Colpo is from............... oh my gosh......Australia!......... I admit that we native born and educated Americans were taught very little about all those 'other' countries out there. In school we did learn that Australia is full of kangaroos and aborigines; however, it wasn't until that specific episode of *The Simpsons* when Homer et al. traveled to Australia that I got to see Aussies in action in their parliament firsthand.

Does this last paragraph seem to be overly cynical and ridiculous? It should. Could there be some correlation between the lackadaisical approach to teaching world geography at the grade school level and the lackadaisical approach of many research professionals in interpreting the actual results of sooooo many studies involving the lipid hypothesis? Although the previous paragraph was written in jest, the thought is frightening.

What is even more frightening regarding that

previous paragraph is that it follows the same unwritten guidelines that many of the medical research studies follow, especially if sponsored by an interest group. I am referring to 'consensus' and 'source'. First, an American 'consensus' that all natives of any faraway country inhabited by aborigines and kangaroos are primitive, confirmed by the 'source' -- Lisa Simpson, the rational genius of the Simpson clan. It is insignificant that Lisa Simpson is animated. She is a 'source' and represents a 'consensus'.

Why then would I blindly follow health advice of a non-doctor like Anthony Colpo? The reason is simple. If I had to choose one book, and one book only regarding what causes heart disease, and more importantly, what does NOT cause heart disease, it would be his *The Great Cholesterol Con*. Although Mr. Colpo is not a doctor, perhaps someday a broadminded university will indeed bestow on him an honorary doctorate degree for his superb independent research in such an important field.

Both Dr. Grisanti and Mr. Colpo take their physical training very seriously. With Dr. Grisanti, it's a family thing. In one of his newsletters, he published a picture of both he and his wife in bathing suits. If there is such a thing as a Mr. and Mrs. America (married) contest, they would be very serious contenders. Mr. Colpo is more modest, and I do not recall seeing a picture of him in a bathing suit; however, according to his neck circumference, it definitely appears that he takes his personal physical training VERY seriously. As a certified fitness professional, he personally pumps the iron big time. The bottom line -- both Dr. Grisanti and Mr. Colpo are diehard advocates of purposeful physical activity for maintaining good health.

I personally have never cared for the gym surroundings for working out -- the loud music, the 'stench' despite the air conditioners working full force.

Esty does like working out at the gym. She also has an interesting observation regarding the difference between the men and women that come to the gym to work out. Men come already stinky to the gym because they will be showering after the workout anyway. Women come to the gym already after a shower and smelling nice......

No, I prefer strength workouts that I can do at home. I don't exercise because I expect to compete in some Olympic strength event. I simply want to stay fit. My preference is isometric or isometric/isotobic type exercises. Isometric workouts are based on exerting a maximum force against an immovable object. This is in contrast to an isotonic type exercise, such as lifting barbells. Isotobic exercise is similar to isometric, only the immovable object is pressing back.

Isometric exercises have been with us for quite a while, even before the name isometric was actually coined. The inventor of modern-day isometric exercise was someone born in 1893 named Angelo Siciliano. Never heard of him? You probably know him by the name of Charles Atlas, crowned the world's most perfectly developed man in the years 1922 and 1923; his isometric exercise method was registered as dynamic tension®.

Anyone growing up in the fifties and sixties who read comic books like I did always saw his advertisements appearing before or after the ads 'Learn to be a locksmith' on the front or back inside covers. Charles Atlas indeed was a 97-pound weakling; the episode where the skinny guy gets sand kicked in his face was based on his real life story.[216]

Charles Atlas rose to fame well before sports, all sports, including bodybuilding, were tainted by anabolic steroid usage. Charles Atlas was natural; he was pure. Testosterone was not synthesized until the 1930's; it was not introduced into the sporting arena until the 1940's and 1950's. Today with the wide use of anabolic steroids, there are no doubt bodybuilders who are bigger and stronger than Charles Atlas; however, none will ever reach his immortality.

It's almost like comparing Barry Bonds to Babe Ruth. Bonds has already surpassed Ruth's total homerun tally; as this is being submitted for printing, he is now very, very close to catching Hank Aaron. Bonds' name has been tainted by possible forbidden drugs usage. Ruth, however, would sign autographs; he visited kids in the hospital; he played ball with kids in the street. Babe Ruth remains a legend. Charles Atlas also remains a legend.

2007

A study published in the April edition of Medicine & Science in Sports & Exercise[217] confirms all the previous conclusions regarding HIIT. Maximum oxygen uptake is considered to be the most important factor determining success in aerobic endurance sports. In this study, subjects were split up into four groups.

1. Long slow distance running (LSD) – 70% of maximum heart rate (HR)
2. Lactate threshold running (LT) – 85% of maximum HR
3. 15/15 interval running – 47 repetitions of 15 seconds intervals, 90-95% of maximum HR

with 15 seconds of rest of 70% max HR
4. 4 X 4 min interval running – 4 intervals of 4 minutes at 90-95% HRmax with 3 min of rest at 70%

The results:

The high-aerobic intensity training performed by the 15/15 and 4x4 min groups increased absolute VO_{2max} significantly compared with the LSD and LT training. Between the 15/15 and the 4 X 4 min groups, no significant difference in training response was observed.

15

What Really are Degenerative Diseases?

The illiterate of the 21st century will not be those who cannot read and write, but those who cannot learn, unlearn, and relearn.
Alvin Toffler

Cardiovascular diseases account for more than half of total mortality before the age of 75 in industrialized countries.[218] Merriam-Webster defines disease as 'a condition of the living animal or plant body or of one of its parts that impairs normal functioning and is typically manifested by distinguishing signs and symptoms'. Most of us equate the term 'disease' with what is properly known as 'infectious disease'.

Infectious diseases result from the activities of microorganisms (living creatures) such as viruses, bacteria, and fungi that invade the body. Influenza, Tuberculosis, Malaria, Measles, Syphilis, Rabies, Smallpox and Polio are

155

examples of infectious diseases. Vaccines and other medications are the tools of the trade in combating infectious diseases.

Heart disease is not an infectious disease. It is defined as a 'degenerative disease'. It is not caused by live microorganisms invading our bodies. I have yet to hear of someone receiving a 'vaccination' against heart disease.

What then is the definition of degenerative disease? The National Cancer Institute defines degenerative disease as 'a disease in which the function or structure of the affected tissues or organs changes for the worse over time'. Simple, right?

Melinda Meade and Robert Earickson in *Medical Geography* define degenerative disease not as a point-blank definition, but rather in terms of its **characteristics**; 'degenerative diseases are *characterized* by the deterioration or impairment of an organ or the structure of cells and the tissues of which they are a part'.

I will concentrate on two particular definitions that I feel zero in on what degenerative diseases really signify. The first is a superb non-technical definition coined by Dr. Ruza Bogdanovich in *The Cure is the Cause*.

> *Degenerative disease occurs when the body does not get what it needs. When it doesn't, it degenerates.*

Another definition appears in Wikipedia:

> *A degenerative disease is a disease in which the function or structure of the affected tissues or organs will progressively deteriorate over time, whether due to normal bodily wear or **lifestyle***

choices such as ***exercise*** or ***eating habits.*** (Bold
emphasis is mine.)

Lifestyle choices!   Exercise and eating habits!
Eating habits entail, of course, food choices. And what is
food exactly?   According Merriam-Webster, food is
'material consisting essentially of protein, carbohydrate,
and fat used in the body of an organism to sustain growth,
repair, and vital processes and to furnish energy'.
    There is nothing negative regarding this definition of
food. Sure, we eat food to supply us with energy, but if
what we eat impairs growth, repair and vital processes, why
then do we still call it 'food'? It should be called 'anti-
food'. Food does not cause degenerative diseases, anti-
food does. The mass of anti-food that you can buy in most
supermarkets is mind-boggling!
    Modern medical technology has indeed found
medical solutions to keep us going when we develop
'degenerative diseases'.
    I arrived that one Friday afternoon to Hadassah
Hospital in the midst of a heart attack, had an additional
two attacks that night while still hooked up to all of the
intravenous infusions. Sunday morning I had a stent
implanted and first thing Monday morning I was already
back on my feet, planning my recovery and return to
normal routine. That is fantastic medical technology.
Future side effects and additional medications aside, it is
still a very impressive feat of technology.
    The bypass operation is another favorite tool used by
cardiology surgeons. Executed for the first time by Dr.
René G. Favaloro at the Cleveland Clinic in 1967,[219]
bypass operations are now very commonplace the world

over. The term itself also brings back fond memories, but not related in any way to heart surgery.

A month before my 17th birthday, I passed my driving test. The routine was receiving a learner's permit, and having an adult family member teach you how to drive in the family car. Our family car at the time was an old 1956 Ford Station Wagon sporting a 292 cubic inch engine. This was the same engine used in the new small two-seater sports car, the Ford Thunderbird. In that big station wagon, it was a powerful engine; those early sporty T-birds must have really flown! Yep, that Ford was big, blue and..... rusty. (I bet you thought I was about to say big, blue and beautiful.)

This was a time when my fellow students would arrive to do their driving test in the new smaller compact cars -- the Chevy Corvair, Ford Falcon and the like. Truthfully, doing parallel parking or the three-point turn-around with a small, and possibly automatic transmission car was a big plus. Looking back, I guess the DMV tester gave me some extra points for showing up to do the test in an 11-year-old huge blue tank with the three-speed manual transmission on the column. I passed the test on my first try.

Sometime after the test, when the old engine was all gummed up on the inside, the oil wasn't circulating from the bottom crankcase to the top of the engine. This caused the car to overheat and lose even more oil. Mechanics then were creative; possibly they received inspiration from their medical colleagues.

The solution: a set of copper 'bypass' pipes connecting the bottom crankcase to the head of the engine. At the time we were so impressed with the recent heart bypass process that whenever anyone asked us what those strange copper pipes were on our engine, we proudly answered that the car had a bypass operation, just like they do now on real people.

Cars are mechanical and made out of metal. There is a natural non-renewable deterioration of the materials and moving parts over time. It is natural for a car to develop a 'degenerative disease'. It is not necessarily natural for us humans, especially before old age.

Cancer is another example of a 'degenerative' disease. Like heart disease, cancer also has its technological solutions. The cardiologist has angioplasty, stent implantation and bypass operations in his bag of tricks. The oncologist has at his disposal chemotherapy, radiotherapy and surgery. These are all 'fixes'. We hear all the time about all the efforts being made to find the 'cure' for cancer.

Well over a half a century ago, Nobel Prize Laureate* Otto Heinrich Warburg discovered that cancer is caused by impaired cell respiration due to a lack of oxygen at the cellular level. This in turn results in hyper-acidity at the same cellular level. Dr. Wigmore cured her own cancer by lifestyle changes, which included a diet more alkaline that acidic. In the 1980's, Dr. Keith Brewer[220] successfully treated patients with various cancers using Cesium, nature's most alkaline mineral, not with radiotherapy and chemotherapy.

---

* Otto Warburg was awarded the 1931 Nobel Prize in Physiology or Medicine. It is believed he was selected for a second Nobel Prize in 1944, but as a Jew was not allowed to accept the prize due to the policies of the German Nazi government at the time. This has never been confirmed by The Nobel Foundation.

What do heart disease and cancer, two degenerative diseases, have in common? Cardiology and oncology researchers spend tremendous resources on improving the 'fixes'; the direction should instead be on 'prevention'. Prevention for both in many cases is feeding the body foods as nature intended, and eliminating the junk that overly taxes the body's ability to digest it. Dr. Maynard Murray was quoted in M.D. Magazine as saying:

> *... the human race is very much what it eats, and if we would pay a bit more attention to the quality of what goes into our mouths, we might be able to find some solutions to two of mankind's more pressing health problems – cancer and arteriosclerosis*

I humbly submit my own supplement to Dr. Bogdanovich's definition of degenerative disease.

> Degenerative disease occurs when the body gets what it doesn't need. When it does, it degenerates.

16

Angiogram #2

February 2007

Chronologically, this is the natural continuation following Chapter 3, which ended with 'to be continued…'. This is the continuation. I did want to review some basic knowledge before reverting back to my personal story. It has been over five and a half years since my heart attack in July 2001. The angiogram performed at that time determined that my main LAD artery (Left Anterior Descending coronary artery) suffered from a blockage of 90%. A blood clot that was unable to navigate the blocked artery was basically the essence of my heart attack. Angioplasty (ballooning) was performed and a stent was installed in the blocked area to keep the artery open.

Two days before my scheduled second angiogram, I arrived at the hospital for the pre-angiogram blood tests and checkup. The doctor performing the checkup asked me the usual questions. Has there been chest discomfort? Do I exercise? She also asked me a question that really took me by surprise. "How many angiograms have you already gone through in the past?"

What bothered me at the time was the intonation in the doctor's voice that this was a typical routine question. It has always been my impression that angiograms are not procedures that people would do routinely many times -- silly me! I answered, "This will be my second time." She recorded the answer and continued with the next question.

Two days after that pre-checkup, I was back on the angiogram table in order to discover and correct the cause of the marginal results of my latest stress test and the subsequent positive results of the thallium heart scan. I had not been experiencing any chest discomfort. Even my professor of cardiology said the angiogram may show the need for a quick, minor correction only, and possibly not even that.

After all, I was feeling great. I had been slowly but surely making vast improvements in my eating habits, and was still considered to be very physically active (bike riding) for my age group. I was well past the initial period when most cases of restenosis (stent blockage) with the standard non-coated stents occur (or so I thought).

The results of the angiogram not only totally surprised me, but my professor of cardiology as well. The stent was totally blocked up -- not a 90% artery blockage like in 2001, however, a full 100%. For two and a half hours, the doctors performing the angiogram tried without success to perform an angioplasty and open up the blockage.

This entire episode raised a number of perplexing questions and uncertainties regarding future action to be taken.

Aren't there usually warning signs of some type when this occurs -- chest pains? fatigue? something? Interestingly, the literature shows that 40% of patients with restenosis may be free of chest pain.[221] According to my cardiologist, the discontinuation of the statins played a critical role. A stent is nevertheless not naturally found in human arteries. Is its closing up somehow concerned with a possible natural body defense mechanism? Didn't my improving eating habits and serious approach to exercising influence this process at all? Did the rest of my arteries suffer similar advancing blockages, or was the problem localized to the stent area only?

How was it I was 'still alive' and fully functioning with a 100% blockage in this critical artery? Will I now need an emergency bypass operation? Medical terminology has another way of referring to a totally blocked artery. It is known as Chronic Total Occlusion (CTO). It was explained to me that while the stent was slowly closing up (probably over the last couple of years) my cardiovascular system was developing new alternative blood vessels (collaterals) to circumvent the constantly narrowing main artery.

Amazing -- my own in-house bypass operation! Many people, the lucky ones not experiencing sudden death, require immediate emergency bypass surgery when this occurs. An immediate ultrasound performed while still on the angiogram table showed that this was unnecessary for me. Why was I one of the lucky ones? Was this due to all the bike riding I do? Improved eating habits? NOT taking statin medication?

And exactly how well are *my* new collaterals functioning. When Chronic Total Occlusion occurs, well-developed collaterals may provide flow equivalent to a 90-

95% stenosis[222] (equivalent to a 90-95% blockage of the original occluded artery). Is this sufficient?

As far as my doctors are concerned this is even more reason to take statins, to protect these new delicate blood vessels. Am I being naive or in self-denial, telling myself that in a sense my own cardiovascular system has performed a sort of internal bypass operation and that I can continue worry free with the status quo? What about the rest of my arteries; are they progressively blocking up also?

I mentioned in SASHA that I was verbally informed back in 2001 that there were additional blockages in my arteries; however, only that one specific blockage in the critical LAD artery required medical intervention. I never received the 2001 angiogram report. My official hospitalization then was at the Mount Scopus branch of Hadassah Hospital; angiograms, angioplasty and such are performed at Hadassah Hospital's Ein Kerem branch.

My present angiogram was done on a Thursday. I was discharged from the hospital Friday morning, a day most offices are already closed for the weekend. First thing Sunday morning, the first day of the normal work week in Israel, I went back to the hospital to see if I could get a copy of that 2001 angiogram report for comparative reasons. I did find the appropriate department, my personal identity information was typed into the terminal, and I could see the report being printed out on the office printer.

This was an exciting moment for me. Besides the 100% blocked stent, has the overall cardiovascular condition of my arteries deteriorated since 2001? Have I been on a 'good path' these last couple of years or simply have I been very, very foolish? In a few seconds I would know.

17

Vindication

*We can't solve problems by using the same kind of
thinking we used when we created them.*
Albert Einstein

T his chapter is actually a natural part of the previous
chapter, however, for me it is of prime importance.
It may be a very short chapter, but the personal
significance of this chapter for me is overwhelming, and
therefore it stands as a separate independent entity.

I compared the 2001 angiogram report with the fresh
2007 one. With the exception of the total restenosis in
2007 (100% stent blockage), **the same partially blocked
locations and the percentage of those blockages in 2001
were identical to the present blockages -- my overall
condition had not worsened**.

2001 Angiogram report

גיל החולה 51.

צינתור שמאלי נערך ביום 15/07/2001 עם שימוש בצנתרים Judkins right 6F , Judkins left 6F .

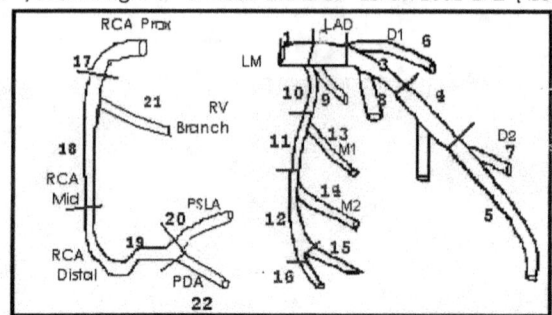

המימצאים בעורקים הכליליים

העורק השמאלי הראשי תקין, מערכת LAD ראה פירוט, מערכת CIRC ראה פירוט, מערכת RCA ראה פירוט.

שם ומספר הסגמנט	מיקום	דרגת קוטר ואומ	זרימה קולטרלית	אפיונים למיקטע	מתאים
		היצרות מ"מ 3- 0	מאין איכות	לבלון לניתוח	
1- LEFT MAIN	תקין				○ ○
4-LAD mid	> 90%				⊙ ○
12-CIRC distal	קל				○ ○
14-Second Marginal	50-70%				○ ○
18-RCA mid	קל ·				○ ○

2001 -Translation:

Name and Segment No.	Degree of Blockage
4 – LAD mid	>90% (angioplasty necessary)
12 – CIRC distal	Light
14 – Second Marginal	50-70%
18 – RCA mid	Light

Vindication

2007 Angiogram report

גיל החולה 57.

צינתור שמאלי נערך ביום 01/02/07 עם שימוש בצנתרים Judkins right 6F , Judkins left 6F .

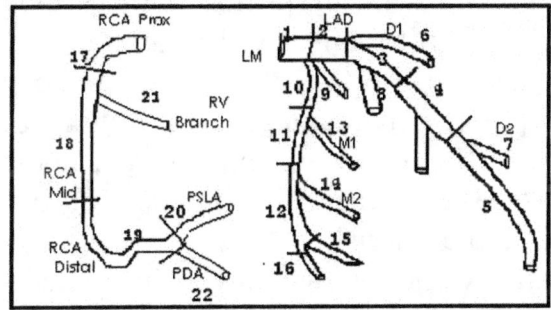

המימצאים בעורקים הכליליים

העורק השמאלי הראשי תקין, מערכת LAD ראה פירוט, מערכת CIRC ראה פירוט, מערכת RCA ראה
פירוט. העורק הימני דומיננטי.

שם ומספר הסגמנט	מיקום	דרגת היצרות מ"מ 3- 0	קוטר ומאי	זרימה קולטרלית		אפיונים למיקטע	מתאים לבלון לניתוח
				מאין	איכות		
4-LAD mid	100%					prox to stent	◯ ⊙
14-Second Marginal	50-70%						◯ ◯
18-RCA mid	קל						◯ ◯

2007 - Translation:

Name and Segment No.	Degree of Blockage
4 – LAD mid – prox to stent	100% (angioplasty necessary)
14 – Second Marginal	50-70%
18 – RCA mid	Light

After three and a half years without the statins and
not being on a low-fat low-cholesterol agenda, the
angiograms did not indicate any significant deterioration in
my artery condition. There was even a light blockage (12–
CIRC distal) that showed up in 2001 that was deemed
insignificant enough not to state in 2007.

167

This was a tremendous relief to me -- a vindication that my eating/exercising habits were indeed keeping the condition of my arteries from deteriorating further. I brought this up with my professor of cardiology who said that really doesn't really confirm anything; the angiogram looks at the inside of the arteries only and certainly doesn't measure possible hardening or thickening of the arteries. This may be a valid point; however, it doesn't negate the fact that I have succeeded in maintaining the status quo -- and without the statins!

I also wonder how many of his patients that come in for the '15-minute' tune up to balloon stents from time to time also take statins, and still need the ballooning. After all, the stent still remains a foreign metal object implanted in a very critical area. One of the functions of cholesterol is to 'bandage' inflamed/damaged arteries. This is a natural defensive action that our bodies perform. The body's natural tendency to insulate the stent from its surroundings is a defensive mechanism.

Chronic total occlusions are found in approximately one-third of the patients with significant coronary disease who undergo angiography.[223] There are three accepted options for dealing with the options available to anyone suffering from Chronic Total Occlusion (CTO).[224]

One option is Percutaneous Intervention, or as more commonly known, angioplasty treatment. Recanalization of a CTO is attempted in only 8-15% of patients undergoing angioplasty.[225] As stated before, this attempt was not successful on me.

The presence of a CTO is a common reason for referral to a second option[226] - coronary artery bypass surgery (CABG). But even a successful bypass operation does not promise a lasting solution. Sections of blood vessels used to create detours around the original blockages tend to develop clogs five to ten years after a bypass.[227] While I realize that a bypass operation is a potential reality for me, I hope to be able to avoid one. In addition, nearly a quarter of the million patients a year who need stents have had bypass surgery in the past.[228] I already have one stent. I really do not want another one.

A third option is described simply as 'medical management'. Bring on the Beta-blockers, ACE-inhibitors, and in particular, the statins. I've gone that route before also. That is basically what SASHA was all about.

In my particular situation, it is imperative to encourage the development of additional blood vessel generation and promote adequate blood flow in my existing cardiovascular system; this is especially true due to the fact that test results show that I am not functioning 100% at the higher heart stress rates. The bottom line, and an agonizing question for me, do I now have to consider the statins in the terms of personal profit and loss?

Dr. Uffe Ravnskov in his pioneering epic *The Cholesterol Myths* acknowledged the cardio health benefits of statins[229] and explained why they are independent of their cholesterol-lowering properties. The statins inhibit the production of a substance called mevalonate, which is a precursor of cholesterol. As mevalonate production decreases, so does cholesterol production. However, mevalonate is also a precursor of other substances in the body that control other important biological functions, some which influence arterial health.

Today there is no doubt that statins do have a beneficial effect on the cardiovascular system. Statins can impair or reverse atherosclerotic plaque formation; improve arterial function; has anti-clotting, anti-inflammatory and antioxidant effects; and prevents atherosclerotic plaque rupture.[230] Cost vs. benefit. I remember all too well my personal costs of the low cholesterol levels caused by the statins.

I respectfully submit my own variation to this third option of 'medical management'. In place of the medications (ESPECIALLY statins), a change in food choices and adequate exercise, the subject of the next chapter.

18

Bottom Line

Off the shelf may be great for software,
but not for your stomach[*]

Food

Anyone from my generation remembers the Watergate scandal during President Nixon's administration and the list of the stars involved. One of the stars was G. Gordon Liddy. He was one tough cookie. It was Liddy's refusal to talk about his role in the Watergate scandal that sent him to prison for a longer term than any other Watergate figure. Time Magazine, in its April 21, 1980 issue, printed some excerpts from his then recent autobiography *Will*.

Then I got the idea for a test to destroy forever
any dread I might still harbor for rats. For the

---

[*] I made that up

next hour, I roasted the dead rat. With a scout knife I skinned, then cut off and ate the roasted haunches of the rat.

For some strange reason, I had always remembered a response that appeared in the Letters to the Editor from a reader who stated:

To G. Gordon Liddy's self-imposed requirement to eat a roasted rat and his activities as an adult, I can only remark, **"You are what you eat.**"[231] (Bold emphasis is mine.)

Yes, we are what we eat. Not only is this a literal expression, but it also now used figuratively as well. The point I am making is both literally and figuratively, *live* people should make an effort to eat more *live* food. Eating only dead food should be seen as expediting the trip to the next whatever-it-is that awaits us all, whether it be a shorter lifespan due to 'natural causes' or an abrupt exit due to some degenerative disease.

My standard breakfast

My basic 'appetizer' is a shot/half a glass of freshly squeezed wheatgrass juice. However on a non everyday schedule which I will discuss shortly, I precede this by dissolving a teaspoon of freshly ground turmeric root in a glass of water. Turmeric has been used for thousands of years to treat a variety of diseases. The active substance in turmeric is curcumin. Curcumin reduces inflammation (a major cause of atherosclerosis) and is also a powerful antioxidant[232] (reduces free radicals).

I follow that with a 'Mike Shlush' (modified Victoria smoothie from chapter 11). I also grind in one clove of garlic (high sulfur content) and ginger (strong free radical scavenging property and known for its anti-inflammatory properties[233]).

I then have my own variation of the Budwig drink. Dr. Johanna Budwig, a German biochemist and multiple Nobel award nominee did extensive research on the properties and benefits of Essential Fatty Acids (EFA's) combined with sulfurated proteins in the diet. Sulfur is a mineral that has the ability to carry oxygen in the body.

Her basic Budwig tonic is based on blending low-fat cottage cheese (or yogurt) with flax seed oil and/or freshly ground flax seeds. When flax seed oil and sulfur-rich protein are combined, the EFA's in the flax seed oil become water-soluble and electron-rich. This increases the stability of the cell membrane and facilitates the transfer of materials and energy between the inner and outer cell membrane.[234] It was her contention that such oils should be consumed together with foods containing the appropriate proteins; otherwise the oils will cause more harm than good.

We saw in Chapter 9 that most of the plaque clogging our arteries is composed of polyunsaturated fats that we consume in our diet. Essential Fatty Acids are polyunsaturated fatty acids that our bodies cannot produce and must be consumed in our diets as polyunsaturated fats.

Nutritionists will come up with different, if not outright conflicting recommendations regarding absolute minimum and maximum requirements. I too have my sources which I choose to accept.

Anthony Colpo mentions that polyunsaturated fats should comprise no more than 4.5% of our total daily calorie intake.[235] Dr. Mary Enig, a world-renowned biochemist specializing in the nutritional aspects of fats and oils, has coauthored many articles with Weston A. Price Foundation head Ms. Sally Fallon Morell. Dr. Enig recommends that we take in at least 2 to 3% of our calories as fat in the form of omega-6 fatty acids and at least 1 to 1.5% in the form of omega-3 fatty acids.[236]

My variation of the Budwig drink:

Instead of yogurt, I use my homemade kefir. I should point out that Dr. Budwig did not specifically mention kefir; it is my own substitute. I mentioned in Chapter 12, when making kefir, the jar must be shaken one to two times per day. This combines the separating whey back into the mixture. Whey proteins contain sulfur, which in turn contains the amino acids cysteine and methionine. The basis for the Budwig drink is sulfur-rich protein.

The kefir I usually make ferments for 48 hours, however only 24 hours during the hot summer months. The extra fermentation time burns off more of the natural milk sugar.

To the kefir I add several tablespoons of freshly ground flax seeds, which is rich in Omega-3. I prefer to use freshly ground flax seeds and not flax seed oil, because the oils become rancid very easily if not properly cared for. Flax seed oil is found in the refrigerated section of your health store; it should be cold-pressed and packaged in an opaque container.[237] At home it must also be kept refrigerated. Flax seed oil should never be heated[238] (as in cooking and frying). Omega-3 is important; however, if you start developing skin rashes, you may be overdoing it with the flax/oil.

I mix in several drops of borage oil. This is my compensation for the aspirin effect of neutralizing the D6D enzyme that promotes production of the conditional fatty acid GLA. It was also found that administration of relatively small amounts of GLA, (up to 360 mg/day) raises the blood levels of arachidonic acid (AA), which is also an important conditional essential fatty acid.[239] Do not overdose on Essential Fatty Acids. Stay within set maximum limits. It was shown that a very high dose of borage oil over a span of a month and a half enhances platelet aggregation;[240] this is something heart patients should be particularly aware of.

I also add a tablespoon of cocoa. Cocoa flavanols may lower inflammation, keep blood pressure in check and prevent platelets from clotting.[241] Cocoa is also a good source of copper. Remember Dr. Klevay and copper deficiency from SASHA?

One third to one half of a teaspoon of fish oil meets requirements for the daily intake of EPA and DHA.[242]

I also add several almonds and walnuts that have been pre-soaked and rinsed.[243] I then add several tablespoons of raw (non-toasted) oat flakes that have also been pre-soaked[244] in whey (phytates and anti-nutrients, remember?). Keep in mind that whole grains are acidic in nature.[245] Slightly aged whey is considered to be a weak acid. Germinating/soaking the grains in an acid medium[246] makes them more alkaline.[247] This reaction is termed 'alkaline-forming' foods.

For 'dessert', I usually have a soft-boiled egg. I buy only organic 'free range' eggs. The nutritional quality of eggs is a function of the food the hens eat. Organic 'free range' eggs have a more balanced healthier omega-3 to omega-6 fatty acid ratio (chapter 9) than commercially grown indoor caged hens. In addition, the eggs of outdoor free range hens are rich in Vitamin D.

My lunch or supper is typically a big salad with meat, fish, or chicken.

My third meal is generally another glass of kefir, and one or more cream cheese (Chapter 12) sandwiches. I no longer make my own baked whole wheat–rye bread as I used to. I now opt for unbaked 'flat bread' made in a food dehydrator. For a great introduction on the use of food dehydrators and illustrated (non wheat) bread recipe, check out 'Igor's Live Flat Bread' by Igor Boutenko - that's right, Victoria's (raw-food) husband. I also use Igor's recipe as the basis of my own variations, such as oat bread/crackers.

During the day I will also 'snack'. Snacks include having another egg or some fruit ('sour' fruits such as apple/grapefruit, and later a sweet fruit such as a banana). I will also drink a glass or two of rejuvelac (chapter 11) if I have some on hand.

Good rules to live by: stay off of sweets, sugars (ESPECIALLY fructose) and white flour as much as possible! Canola oil still does NOT enter my household. I realize that it is still a favorite with 'heart' dieticians because it is a mono-unsaturated oil like olive oil. Anything you need to know about Canola oil can be found on the Weston A. Price website.

I have said it before, but I will say it again -- eliminate totally all partially hydrogenated ingredients from your diet. *THE* Internet site on partially hydrogenated oils and trans-fats is Stephen Joseph's www.bantransfats.com[*].

---

[*] See how you can get your own 'Don't partially hydrogenate me' T-shirt and bumper sticker!

Statins (HMG CoA reductase inhibitors)

Immediately following my two-and-a-half-hour angiogram, I took another look at the short-term benefits vs. costs of taking statins. I did decide to resume a hydrophilic statin[**] temporarily -- for four weeks and taper off by the sixth week. This was not to lower my cholesterol levels, but rather for other short-term effects which may be specifically beneficial for me after getting 'poked at from within' on the angiogram table, i.e. anti-inflammatory effects, anti-clotting, prevention of plaque rupture[248] etc. Statin therapy does appear to reduce the incidence of stroke, myocardial infarction, and death within 30 days after angioplasty and stent placement.[249] However, this time I also took coenzymeQ_{10} with it - not because my doctor told me, but because of all the evidence that statins deplete the body of coenzymeQ_{10}.

Warning:
HMG CoA reductase inhibitors block the endogenous biosynthesis of an essential cofactor, coenzymeQ_{10}, required for energy production. A deficiency of coenzymeQ_{10} is associated with impairment of myocardial function, with liver dysfunction and with myopathies (including cardiomyopathy and congestive heart failure). ***All patients taking HMG CoA reductase inhibitors should therefore be advised to take***

[**]as opposed to a lipophilic statin – for the most up-to-date and complete guide to statin medication, visit Dr. Duane Graveline's website http://www.spacedoc.net

100 to 200mg per day of supplemental coenzymeQ$_{10}$.[250] (Bold emphasis is mine.)

It may have been prudent to also take selenium supplements during this period, but for the limited period I didn't.

We noted that the pattern of side effects associated with statins resembles the pathology of selenium deficiency…… A negative effect of statins on selenoprotein synthesis does seem to explain many of the enigmatic effects and side effects of statins, in particular, statin-induced myopathy (muscular weakness)[251]

I stated previously that I am functioning normally in spite of the blocked main artery due to the generation of new blood vessels which circumvented my blocked stent. Let's take a closer look at what I referred up until now as simply 'new blood vessels'.

Angiogenesis

Angiogenesis is a process by which new capillary blood vessels sprout from a preexisting blood vessels. Stated more scientifically, it is a process in which endothelial cells proliferate and differentiate to form a fine capillary tree.

Capillaries are designed to provide maximum nutrient delivery efficiency. A greater number of capillaries also allows for greater oxygen exchange in our bodies. The driving force for angiogenesis is ischemia[252] (restriction in blood supply, generally due to factors in the smaller blood vessels). Angiogenesis is also induced by hypoxia[253] (shortage of oxygen). Hypoxia would be a natural consequence resulting from ischemia.

Angiogenesis, however, has not been shown to be correlated with increased blood flow,[254] (angiogenesis is not compensation for an occluded artery) which brings us to our next term:

Arteriogenesis

Arteriogenesis is the rapid proliferation of preexisting standby collateral arteries known as arterioles; it refers to an increase in the diameter of existing arterial vessels. Newly generated arteries can expand up to 20 times the diameter of the original arteriole.[255] In principle this mechanism resembles a deflated bicycle inner tube that stays flat until needed. When pumping it up with physical force, the once flat, airless inner tube becomes an expanding diameter air-filled tube.

Mechanically, arteriogenesis is linked to elevated pressure (physical force). This in turn increases radial wall stress, and fluid shear stress (elevated flow), which increases endothelial surface stress. Chronically elevated fluid shear stress was found to be the strongest trigger of arteriogenesis under experimental conditions.[256]

As I have personally experienced, it is possible to functionally replace an occluded (blocked) artery completely by collaterals.[257]

The most basic differences between angiogenesis and arteriogenesis are summarized on the following chart:[258]

	Angiogenesis	Arteriogenesis
Initiated by	Ischemia (blockage)	Shear Stress
Substrate	Preexisting capillaries	Preexisting arterioles
Result	Increased capillary density	New arteries
Time	Days	Days to weeks

Obviously, angiogenesis and arteriogenesis are terms that have taken on a new significance for me. In this regard, will statins be beneficial for me? Studies indicate that statins have a biphasic potential either to promote or inhibit angiogenesis. Low statin doses induce a pro-angiogenic effect, and high statin doses cause an anti-angiogenic effect.[259]

Studies are great for the researchers, but for us patients what does this really mean? Are the current doses in clinical use that we humans take pro-angiogenic or anti-angiogenic? This was a question I put to a number of researchers. An answer that I received is 'current doses in clinical use are probably pro-angiogenic, however, this remains an educated guess.' As I learned from my two-year, 20mg Pravastatin period, not all patients have the same tolerance to medication as others. What may be a low dose for someone could very well be a high dose for someone else. Let's assume for the argument that it is indeed pro-angiogenic in most cases. Is that a good thing or a bad thing? For a damaged area of the heart, it may be a very good thing; however, does this mean that artificially stimulated angiogenesis is good for the body as a whole? The National Cancer Institute states[260] that:

> *Cancer spreads by metastasis, the ability of cancer cells to penetrate into lymphatic and blood vessels, circulate through the bloodstream, and then invade and grow in normal tissues elsewhere....* *Cancer researchers studying the conditions necessary for cancer metastasis have discovered that one of the critical events required is the growth of a new network of blood vessels. This process of forming new blood vessels is called* **angiogenesis.** (Bold emphasis is mine.)

Dr. Judah Folkman stated as early as 1971 that cancer tumors were angiogenesis-dependent.[261] Dr. Napoleone Ferrara stated straight to the point and very bluntly:

> *Abnormal regulation of angiogenesis has been implicated in the pathogenesis of several disorders, including cancer.*[262]

Angiogenesis? I prefer to depend on my own body chemistry to regulate my angiogenesis rate by natural means. Am I being overly panicky? With regards to statins and their relationship to cancer:

- *Use of cholesterol-lowering drugs should be restricted to those at high risk of short-term CHD death, such as those with prior CHD.*[263]

- *A disturbing increased incidence of cancers has been reported in two randomized controlled trials of the hydrophilic 3- hydroxy-3-methylglutaryl CoA (HMG-CoA) reductase inhibitor pravastatin—Prospective Study of Pravastatin in the Elderly at Risk (PROSPER;ref.1) and Cholesterol and Recurrent Events (CARE;ref.2). In the PROSPER[*] trial, the reduction in deaths from vascular events was completely negated by the increase in deaths from cancer. In the CARE trial, breast cancer occurred in a significantly greater number of women treated with pravastatin.......**There is clearly an urgent need for further controlled trials of the individual statins with inclusion of cancer mortality as a clinical end point.**[264]*
  (Bold emphasis is mine.)

- *Squalene, the immediate precursor to cholesterol, has anti-cancer effects, according to research.[265]*

I mentioned previously that I grind up a teaspoon of the spice turmeric in the morning – but not every morning. The active ingredient in turmeric is curcumin, which has been shown to be an inhibitor of angiogenesis. If my primary health concern today was fighting cancer, I probably would take turmeric every morning. Since today I am more concerned with the anti-inflammatory benefits of turmeric, I do not take it every morning in order to

---

[*] CARE and PROSPER were two studies researching the effects of statins on heart disease – the cancer findings were an added surprise.

minimize my own interference in my natural angiogenesis process.[266]

I hope I am wrong, however, my gut feeling tells me the next decade will see a dramatic increase in research studies proving a definite positive correlation between statin usage and an increase in the incidence of cancer.

Will a cancer epidemic overtake the heart disease epidemic as the number one cause of death?

As important that angiogenesis is for small capillary generation, my main concern, due to the stent blockage, is blood flow and arteriogenesis. Do statins affect arteriogenesis positively or negatively? Tests do show that statins improve general arterial function by specifically improving endothelial function.[267]

Interestingly, the positive effects of statins on endothelial function disappear a short time after discontinuation of taking them. A test involving atorvastatin (Lipitor) showed these benefits disappeared in a mere 36 hours. Incidentally, the half-life of atorvastatin is approximately 14 hours, which is about 10 times longer than the half-life of most other statins.[268]

An important regulator of coronary collateral growth is nitric oxide.[269] The statins ability to increase nitric oxide production[270] leads to an increase in Endothelial Progenitor Cells (EPC) and improved endothelial function.[271]

Is there a relationship between the dose of the statins and development of the collaterals? Good question. One study says no[272] (and by the way also specifically states that there is no relationship between collateral development and LDL cholesterol levels). Another study found that collateral development was viable only with statin doses of at least 10mg of atorvastatin or equivalent.[273]

Again, is artificially interfering with production of progenitor cells beneficial or harmful? A 2007 study warns that:

> *caution should be used in the manipulation of circulating progenitor cells for therapeutic strategies.*[274]

A bit confused? You should be; so am I. There is a much better way to increase nitric oxide production and increase circulating Endothelial Progenitor Cells. The answer – EXERCISE! In the last years, several groups were able to show the positive effects of exercise on Endothelial Progenitor Cells.[275]

It has been shown that growth of these collateral arteries is triggered by physical forces, which increases fluid shear stress on the vessels. Fluid shear stress initiates the activation of Endothelial Cells.[276] And as a bonus, shear stress is also known to lead to the release of nitric oxide.[277]

I prefer to increase my nitric oxide production and my circulating EPC's by bike riding rather than by statin popping. Antioxidants (found in nuts and seeds), a little garlic and keeping a lid on sugar also promote nitric oxide (NO) production.[278]

Regarding NO production and arteriogenesis in particular:

> *Maintenance, or improvement, of NO production and signaling, such as with regular exercise, may improve endothelial cell function and thus may help preserve the arteriogenic potential of preexisting collateral networks.*[279]

Statins are the ultimate invention of the twentieth/twenty-first century. For those who cannot, or simply will not exercise by choice, the statin offers a solution, a calculated risk solution. For those who choose not to eat properly the statin does offer an alternative, again, a calculated risk alternative.

What exactly is a calculated risk? When Israeli Prime Minister Ariel Sharon had a minor stroke on December 18, 2005, the cause was attributed to a clot lodged in a small 1 - 2mm hole in his heart. The hole was a minor birth defect, also found in 15-20% of the population.[280] Prime Minister Sharon was given heavy doses of blood-thinning medication, which can be associated with an increased risk of brain hemorrhage; this was the calculated risk. The purpose of this medication was to prevent another occurrence of a clot pending the heart operation. On January 4, 2006, the night before his scheduled heart operation and while still at home, he suffered a major stroke with massive internal bleeding. He has been in a vegetative state ever since.

To statin or not to statin -- that is the question. It comes down to a choice between two alternatives.

I start the day off with a shot of wheatgrass, which I have been growing and nurturing for the last seven to ten days. I make my own personal breakfast cereal which includes homemade kefir; the kefir is made from raw milk that I have to obtain from the 'underground'. It has been fermenting for the last 48 hours and has to be filtered to separate the grains from the liquid. To this I add oats that have been soaking for the last 24 hours in whey (slightly acidic), walnuts and almonds that have been soaking in a salt solution, freshly ground flax seeds, besides other ingredients. I repeat this filtering process for another glass of kefir in the evening. I make my own cheese; total processing time is measured in days. I find the time for daily deliberate physical activity that can range from half an hour to one and a half hours.

Or…….

I can simply take a statin.

For me the choice is obvious. I willingly choose the former. My gripe is that statins are now given as a first-choice method of treatment; due to their disastrous side effects I consider them to be more of a last resort. If, as I grow older and find that for reasons beyond my control I will no longer be able to exercise as much as I believe to be necessary, I will again weigh the costs vs. the benefits of taking statin medication. And even then, the dosage will be much smaller than the accepted clinical dosages prescribed today.[281] For now, I prefer the natural alternatives.

Exercise

While still on the angiogram table, my professor stated that it was probably the bike riding that helped develop my internal bypasses. Indeed, medical studies do confirm that blood vessels enlarge when chronically exposed to high flows.[282] What then would be the ultimate exercise method to maintain these new bypass arteries at an optimal level? Research also shows that once new arteries open up, they also rapidly decrease in size if overall decreased blood flow warrants it (decreased wall stress).[283]

Introducing HIIT (grizzly bear) workouts in my riding routine has allowed me to have an adequate workout, when short of time or when especially poor weather keeps me inside. With all of its benefits for cardiovascular health (chapter 14) is it, however, the best way to promote and maintain arteriogenesis? Is arteriogenesis better served by longer-term moderate exercising? Dr. Ulrich Laufs and associates demonstrated that:

Intensive and moderate exercising for 30 min, but not for 10 min, increased circulating levels of EPC, which may represent an important beneficial outcome of physical exercise.[284]

EPC's (Endothelial Progenitor Cells) are made in the bone marrow, enter the bloodstream and go to areas of blood vessel injury to help repair the damage. The number of circulating Endothelial Progenitor Cells in an individual's blood may be an indicator of overall cardiovascular health.[285] Therefore, depletion and aging (senescence) of EPC's may contribute to blood vessel disease.

All exercise is beneficial, as long as not overdoing it.[286] I have adapted several different bike-riding styles to my riding routine. I try at least once a week to go out for an enjoyable off-road trail ride, which encompasses several hours of all the elements of intensity and duration according to the terrain. I use a pulse meter to regulate my efforts as necessary.

During the week when I am usually more pressed for time, I may do alternating days of HIIT (grizzly bear) workouts; days with longer-duration lower-intensity including steady uphill riding, or simply an enjoyable easy fresh-air ride.

This way I am hopefully benefiting from the best of all worlds -- overall cardiovascular health with an emphasis on arteriogenesis.

The role of the 2-P's in long term exercise planning

The reality of functioning with an occluded artery has reinforced the importance of maintaining a structured riding schedule. As with most other aspects in life, we must work hard to achieve our goals. It takes both persistence and perseverance- the 2 P's - to reach long term goals. For this reason, I want to lump the 2 P's together for the purpose of achieving long term goals as follows:

> Persistence/perseverance is the technique utilized to obtain an ambitious long term goal. A long term goal does not necessarily have a set time deadline. In order to achieve the long term goal, it is divided into a number of short term goals. Each short term goal DOES have a deadline. Moreover, the success or failure of the short term goal must be measurable by some objective method. Persistence/perseverance is the sequence of successfully achieving short term goals over time.

My master long term goal is to maintain the status quo regarding my existing heart disease. This is a *v-e-r-y l-o-n-g t-e-r-m* goal without a set time deadline. One of the means at my disposal to obtain this master goal is to set another smaller *long term* goal WITH a deadline, that involves physical exercise in general, and my bike riding in particular. I have been riding an average 6,000km (3,730mi) per year, and this has become my yearly goal. 6,000km!?! That is further than the air space between New York and Madrid, Spain! Sounds impossible? Even if there was a bridge connecting both sides of the Atlantic Ocean?

As per my 2-P's doctrine, I divide this ambitious long term goal into 52 short term goals, or, my weekly quota. That is more or less the distance of a weekly round-trip bike ride between Baltimore and Washington D.C.; this still sounds ambitious, but not as 'impossible' as riding the distance between New York to Madrid. In order to meet this short term goal, I keep track of the kilometers/miles that I ride each week. An hour to an hour-and-a-half of daily riding allows me to achieve my weekly goal. The sequence of successfully achieving short term weekly goals over time ultimately results in my meeting my annual goal, which is simply the means to the end of maintaining my status quo.

And it works.

The additional payoff of daily riding and keeping in shape allows me to really enjoy my weekend bike treks with family and friends. Pictures from some of my bike trips are posted on my web site (www.heartrecovery.net).

♥ ♥ ♥

I will be very happy when a serious researcher will determine

    1. if there is a greater positive correlation between 'HIIT and arteriogenesis' as

compared to 'longer-duration lower / moderate exercising and arteriogenesis'.

2. if there is any (positive or negative) correlation between HIIT and the cardiovascular health of the specific areas in the arteries that are most susceptible to potential or existing heart disease (areas experiencing the greatest 'sheer stress').[287]

Important tip – when riding in the summer on hot days, be sure to supplement your water with natural salt.[288]

If you are the gym type, then definitely go to the gym. My isometric/isotobic exercise I do at home.

And finally and maybe most important…

And finally and maybe most important…

And finally and maybe most important…

In SASHA, I stated that I considered the heart attack to be a technical temporary setback; I would be back to normalcy in a minimum amount of time. Granted, the statins took me off this timetable for a number of years, but they didn't quell my innermost desire to be 'healthy' again.

Everything up until now stated in this book as been technique only. Proper eating habits and proper exercise are important; however, they are not enough. Anyone who dwells on personal setbacks 'oh I am a miserable unfortunate guy' will always be that, a miserable unfortunate guy. Despite my heart attack, the stent, the total restenosis (blockage) in my main LAD artery, **I am healthy**. No doctor can convince me otherwise!

.

19

Epilogue

To copy one person's work is plagiarism, to copy many, is research

Accoring to this definition from an unknown source, this book is certainly not plagiarism; I have quoted from many other works. Does that qualify it as research? I think not! There is nothing truly original in this book. I have invented nothing. I have collected previously published information that I believe will contribute to keeping my cardiovascular system as healthy as possible for my own personal health benefits. Some of my sources are well known, such as Ms. Sally Fallon Morell and her associates from the Weston A. Price Foundation; Dr. Anne Wigmore and others; some of the other sources are not as well known.

Anyone interested in implementing habits that I have acquired to maintain my cardiovascular health should keep in mind that I attribute my current health status to the complete package I have written about. Anyone deciding to 'simply stop taking statins like Mike did', but is not willing to make necessary changes in diet and invest the necessary effort in physical exercise is only deceiving himself.

It may very well be that only a certain few of the changes I have made are responsible for a significant improvement in health; while the effects of some of the changes may be of marginal value only. Taking the easy road out may be risky and lead to undesirable consequences.

It is also difficult to implement a decision when it contradicts the accepted way of doing things, especially if the decision involves personal health issues. The accepted way of preventing and treating heart disease is keeping cholesterol levels at 'acceptable levels'. The accepted ways of accomplishing this is by keeping to low-fat diets and supplementing the process with medications, i.e. statins. Why? Because as far back as our personal memories go, **that's the way it's always been**. End of story.

An amusing story of unknown origins illustrates this point quite well. It is presented to management training students. The story involves a 'study' of five monkeys in a cage. A banana was hung from the top of the cage and a set of stairs was placed under it. For those unfamiliar with monkeys, they naturally like bananas. Almost immediately a monkey started to climb up the stairs in order to retrieve the banana. As soon as he touched the stairs, all of the other monkeys were sprayed with cold water. After a while, another monkey made an attempt with the same results. All the other monkeys were sprayed with cold water. Ultimately, when any monkey tried to climb the stairs, all the other monkeys prevented him from doing so in order not to get the cold shower.

At this stage the cold shower mechanism was disconnected, then one of the original monkeys was removed from the cage and replaced with a new one. The new monkey saw the banana and dashed to the stairs. To his surprise, all of the other monkeys attacked him. After another attempt and attack, he knew what the consequences would be if he tried to climb the stairs.

Again, another of the original five monkeys was replaced with a new one. The newcomer went for the stairs and was attacked. The previous newcomer participated in the punishment with all the other veterans. Next, a third original monkey was replaced, then the fourth, and finally the fifth. Every time the newest monkey took to the stairs, he was attacked. The newest monkeys that were attacked had no idea why they were not permitted to climb the stairs; they also had no idea why they were participating in the beating of the newest monkey.

After all the original monkeys were replaced, none of them had ever been sprayed with cold water. Nevertheless, no monkey ever again approached the stairs to try for the banana. Why not? Because **that's the way it's always been.**

Man is capable of doing marvelous things. Man has put other men on the moon. Man has built computer chips executing millions of operations per second.

Man is also capable of doing the most heinous acts, the mass murder or mutilation of other human beings. The English language has a term for this; it is called genocide. The term itself was coined by Raphael Lemkin in 1943, from the roots *genos (Greek)* for family, tribe or race) and -*cide* (Latin) - *occidere* or *cideo* - meaning to massacre.

Genocide is defined by the Convention on the

Prevention and Punishment of the Crime of Genocide[289] (CPPCG) Article 2 as:

> *any of the following acts committed with intent to destroy, in whole or in part, a national, ethnic, racial or religious group, as such: Killing members of the group; Causing serious bodily or mental harm to members of the group; Deliberately inflicting on the group conditions of life calculated to bring about its physical destruction in whole or in part; Imposing measures intended to prevent births within the group; and forcibly transferring children of the group to another group.*

Unfortunately, the twentieth century alone, despite all of its technological advances, bore witness to many atrocities. To name just a few:

- 1915-1918: 1,500,000 Armenians slaughtered.
- 1932-33: 7,000,000 perished in Ukraine due to the deliberated caused famine by Joseph Stalin.
- 1938 through 1945: Despite denials by some so-called scholars, as well as several of today's world leaders, the Nazi holocaust DID happen. It was real. Six million Jews perished in the death camps.
- Cambodia: 2,000,000 deaths due to executions, deliberate starvation and overwork - Khmer Rouge leader Pol Pot.
- Rwanda: up to 800,000 Tutsis were killed by Hutu militia using clubs and machetes.

- More recently – the on-going atrocities going in the Darfur region of western Sudan against the non-Arab villagers.

And this horrific list is not all-inclusive.

No doubt, decent people the world over are appalled by these atrocities. But what does one call a non-violent systematic method that kills and maims millions every year?

Medicines to lower blood pressure and bad cholesterol are already effective and widely used, yet heart disease remains the biggest cause of death in the United States, killing 911,000 people in 2003, according to the American Heart Association.[290]

There was nothing exceptional regarding heart disease as the leading cause of death in 2003. In every year since 1900, except 1918, cardiovascular disease accounted for more deaths than any other single cause or group of causes of death in the United States.[291]

Shouldn't the millions and millions of deaths caused by CHD generate the same disgust that death by genocide creates? The data shows that over the last 100 years, with the widespread use of all types of modern manufactured food, including the pasteurized dead milk products and hydrogenated oil products, just to name a few, the rate of mortality due to CHD has almost tripled.

In 1901 in the USA, there were 140 deaths[292] per 100,000 caused by 'diseases of the heart'. This number peaked to 375.5 deaths[293] in 1963 and since then has been tapering off. The medical establishment sees this as verification that it is making headway in stopping heart disease. This is a naive outlook. Although the medical establishment should be commended for making technological advances in improving medical procedures (stents/bypass operations) for saving heart attack victims, heart disease itself is not declining.

Overwhelming evidence proves that the lipid hypothesis is based on bad science. It is not valid. Simply put, it is not the cholesterol or saturated fat that has caused the rate of deaths due to CHD to nearly triple over the last hundred years. This increase occurred in spite of a decline in the saturated fats in the American diet and improved techniques for taking care of heart attack patients over the last 40 years.

Here we get to the crux of the problem. This is no single tyrant, Adolf Hitler or Pol Pot, that can be blamed for this phenomenon of millions dying because of CHD. The industries that for many years were utilizing partially hydrogenated oil in their products, resulting in high trans-fat content, were encouraged and promoted by official U.S. agencies that were established to protect our health. Pasteurization is firmly set by law, the sale and distribution of non-pasteurized milk/products is either outright illegal in most states, or overly restricted.

With no intent to insult the feminist movement, breast-feeding is by far the healthiest and cheapest way to feed babies. Baby formula was the natural response to the higher mortality[294] and higher sickness rate of babies fed pasteurized cow's milk instead of natural mother's milk.

In 1976, it was reported that in a particular Californian city, it cost almost three times as much to buy ready made baby formula as it did to buy food for the nursing mother.[295] Respected multinational companies

actively market expensive substitute milk formulas in ....
Africa... of all places. The cost of purchasing milk
substitutes in many third world countries is a crippling slice
of the monthly salary.[296] This also does not take into
consideration the hidden costs of chronic illnesses and
inferior development of the babies in the future who were
denied mothers' milk.[297]

I mentioned in the beginning of SASHA that I was
never an avid reader; as such I do not possess an especially
rich treasury of words. I was not able to find an existing
word that accurately describes this phenomenon of peaceful
genocide that I want to discuss now. As a result, I am
forced to coin my own term.

Troficide - *trofi (Greek)* for food and *-cide* (Latin)
- *occidere* or *cideo* - meaning to massacre.

I also respectfully submit a definition for this new
term:

Troficide is the systematic nutritional killing or
maiming of humans regardless of national,
ethnic, racial or religious group, as such: Killing
members of the group; Causing serious bodily or
mental harm to members of the group;
Deliberately inflicting on the group conditions of
life calculated to bring about its physical
destruction in whole or in part; and forcibly
transferring children from their mothers' breasts.

Man is capable of doing marvelous things. Man has
put other men on the moon. Man has built computer chips

executing millions of operations per second. Man is also capable of putting an end to 'troficide'.

20

Post-Epilogue

Coexistence... what the farmer does with the turkey
- until Thanksgiving.
Mike Connolly

Here is another one "The only alternative to coexistence is codestruction" - Jawaharlal Nehru. On this optimistic introduction, and with the intent of closing this book on a lighter note and not with 'troficide', I leave you with the following question. How does one half of a couple who needs significant freezer space to freeze fresh raw milk, and additional refrigerator space to cool dripping fresh cheese, bottles of whey, rejuvelac and fermenting sauerkraut, coexist in what is otherwise known as a normal kitchen/household?

Leave it to Esty to come up with a creative solution to my unconventional eating habits. Esty recently surprised me with my very own refrigerator. Yes, you read that correctly. No, it is nowhere as large as the family fridge, and I did have to clean out a corner of a storage room to fit it in; however, it has made sharing the same kitchen 'more pleasant'. No, it was not intended as a present for the 'man who already has everything'.

You can categorize the fridge as the type of present where the 'giver' benefits as much as the 'givee'. I get to buy larger quantities of fresh raw milk at a time, and Esty keeps me out of 'her' freezer!

According to my spellchecker, it appears that I have created another new word, 'givee'. I probably should have used the word 'recipient'.

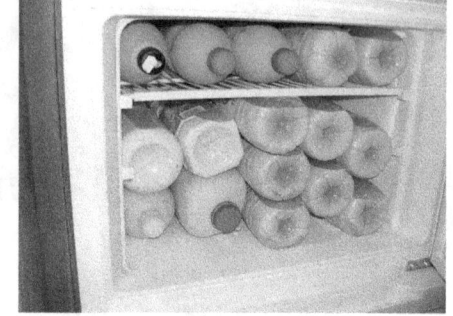

But then again, after the stent and the statins, I have learned to bend the existing rules a bit.

July 13, 2007 3:30 PM

Exactly six years ago today I arrived to Hadassah Hospital in Jerusalem in the midst of a heart attack. Much has occurred in the Stone household over the last six years. When I first started writing this book well over a year ago, I wrote (chapter 2):

> Within six years after a recognized heart attack (MI), 18% of men will have another heart attack, about 22% will be disabled with heart failure, 8% will have a stroke and 7% will experience sudden death.[298]

At the time I was still under the illusion that the 'six-year rule' did not apply to me. Why should it? I had extensively changed my eating and exercise habits. As destiny would have it, I discovered following routine testing that the stent inserted in my critical main artery (LAD) had become 100% clogged -- 100% restenosis.

However, I did *not* have another heart attack; I was *not* disabled with heart failure and did *not* experience sudden death.

Despite this total blockage in such a critical area, a bypass operation in the foreseeable future is not even in the cards. Except for the pinpoint blockage at the stent location (chapter 17), my overall condition has not deteriorated despite my abandoning many of the consensus-accepted rules for coping with/preventing heart disease. You are free to draw your own conclusions.

And for the record, the cats that participated in the 'cat scan' in chapter 7 are all alive, well and smiling.

21

2010

*Discovery consists in seeing what everyone else
has seen and thinking what no one else
has thought.*
Albert Szent-Gyorgyi

Is there such a thing as Post Statin Syndrome (PSS)? In 10 years time, if you google this term, this book might be the only place where the term occurs – or – it may be the most searched for illness in the first part of the 21st century.

There is a myriad of information regarding the negative side effects of statin medication, cognitive problems, memory loss, personality changes, and irritability. Regarding irritability, case studies have demonstrated that

*Manifestations of severe irritability included
homicidal impulses, threats to others, road*

rage, generation of fear in family members, and damage to property.[299]

But what happens AFTER the physical effects subside after the discontinuation of the statins? As I discussed in SASHA, I felt an emotional recovery very shortly after discontinuing the statins in 2003. Dr. Golomb mentioned in her research that cognitive dysfunctions return to pre-statin functioning after approximately 6 months.

What then is Post Statin Syndrome (PSS)? Time is a dynamic entity. It waits for no one. It goes back for no one. Physical, mental and emotional functioning of the individual may revert back to pre-statin levels. However, what about the effect that the statin period has on one's interactions with his/her personal surroundings? To the best of my knowledge, there are no research endeavors of the 'post' statin period. I can only relate what a post statin period looks like from my own personal perspective. I discussed in SASHA my cognitive dysfunction at work. I also mentioned a schism in my relations at home with Esty.

What I didn't delve into at the time was what had occurred with colleagues and co-workers during this period. As I am approaching some forty odd years of gainful employment, I can say that what characterized my interpersonal relationships throughout my work career, was that I truly got along with everyone - superiors, colleagues, subordinates - everyone. During my statin period, I found myself in the strange setting of NOT getting along with superiors, colleagues and subordinates.

I mentioned time is dynamic? Towards the end of 2003, when I was totally weaned off of the negative effects of the statins, my messed up relations with others at work stayed messed up. Maybe if I was of stronger character, I could have been more proactive in trying to mend impaired relations with colleagues, as I was able to accomplish with Esty. But I wonder how many people that get caught up in the statin web never really manage to escape it.

Almost two years after the physical effects of the statins had subsisted, at work I nearly found myself in a physical fight with co-worker almost young enough to be my son. Sure, the guy was an obnoxious bastard and was capable of dissecting me in a physical confrontation.

However we encounter types like this all the time - in stores, on the road, at gas stations, even neighbors. We certainly cannot go around 'slugging' people just because they are obnoxious bastards. In mid 2005, which coincided with two years after getting off the statins, I realized that there was just too much to fix in repairing strained relationships at work. I decided to resign - the final necessary step to seal off my post statin syndrome period. I left a job with a good salary and excellent benefits; I quit for the unknown.

Not fair? If you are at the age where you can list on your curriculum vitae (CV) of life that you have had a heart attack, then you can probably count the decades you have left on this planet with the fingers on one hand. No one is really born with inalienable rights. It's a great campaign slogan for politicians, but that is not how the real world works. Play the cards you are now holding, get on with the rest of your life, and move on. That works for me; I hope it works for you.

References

Chapter 1

1. Benjamin Franklin, Poor Richard's Quotations (1975)

Chapter 2

2. Ignarro L., NO More Heart Disease: How Nitric Oxide Can Prevent -- Even Reverse -- Heart Disease and Stroke, St. Martin's Griffin; 2006, page 31

3. Ravnskov U, The Cholesterol Myths: Exposing the Fallacy that Saturated Fat and Cholesterol Cause Heart Disease NewTrends Publishing, 2000, 50-52

4. Stone M. Surviving a Successful Heart Attack second edition, Lulu, 2005, 30-39

5. Kauffman J. Malignant Medical Myths: Why Medical Treatment Causes 200,000 Deaths in the USA each Year, and How to Protect Yourself, Infinity Publishing, 2006,165

Chapter 3

6. Fuster V et al, Hurst's The Heart, Mcgraw-Hill 2000, 7

Chapter 4

7. Howell E., Enzyme Nutrition, Avery, 1995, xv, 3-5,7,16,33-35,80,123,148,149,154

8. Bairoch A, The Enzyme database in 2000, Nucleic Acids Res 28: 304-305

9. Becker Gh, Meyer J, Necheles H. Fat absorption and atherosclerosis. Science. 1949 Nov 18;110(2864):529

Becker Gh, Meyer J, Necheles H. Fat absorption in young and old age. Gastroenterology. 1950 Jan; 14(1):80-92

10. Pilgeram LO, Deficiencies in the lipoprotein lipase system in atherosclerosis., J Gerontol. 1958 Jan; 13(1):32-42

11. Pottenger FM. Pottenger's Cats: A Study in Nutrition, Price-Pottenger Nutrition Foundation, 1995

12. Pottenger FM, 18

13. MacDonald ML et al. Nutrition of the domestic cat, a mammalian carnivore., Annu Rev Nutr. 1984; 4:521-62

14. Knopf K et al. Taurine: an essential nutrient for the cat., J Nutr. 1978 May; 108(5):773-8

15. Sturman JA et al. Feline maternal taurine deficiency: effect on mother and offspring J Nutr.1986 Apr; 116(4):655-67

16. Fallon S. Nourishing Traditions: The Cookbook that Challenges Politically Correct Nutrition and the Diet Dictocrats Sec ed., NewTrends Publishing 1999, xi xii

17. Pottenger FM, 3

18. Boutenko V et al., Raw Family: A True Story of Awakening, Raw Family, 2000

19. Kroeger H. God helps those that help themselves, Privately printed, 1984, 13, 220

Chapter 6

20. Antoine Béchamp, La Théorie du Microzyma (preface)

21. Douglass WC. The Milk Book: The Milk of Human Kindness Is Not Pasteurized, Rhino Publishing, S.A., 2004, 121

References

22. New York Times, The Doctor's World; Revisionist History Sees Pasteur As Liar Who Stole Rival's Ideas, May 16, 1995

23. Washington Post, USA Today Reporter Resigns Over Probe Thursday, January 8, 2004; Page C01

24. Hume ED. Béchamp or Pasteur? A Lost Chapter in the History of Biology Sec ed., E.W. Daniel Company, 1932, 205

25. Id at 281

26. Lanctôt G. The Medical Mafia: How to Get Out of It Alive and Take Back Our Health & Wealth, Here's the Key 1995, 157

27. Hiestand S&D, Electrical Nutrition: A revolutionary approach to eating that awakens the body. Avery, 2001, 67

28. Pfizer Inc. 2006 Financial Report page 78, Pfizer website http://www.pfizer.com/pfizer/annualreport/2006/financial/p2006 fin79.jsp - viewed May 19, 2007

29. IBID

30. IBID at 16

31. Graveline D. Lipitor Thief of Memory, Infinity, 2004

Chapter 7

32. Douglass WC. 16

33. Schmid R. The Untold Story of Milk: Green Pastures, Contented Cows and Raw Dairy Products, NewTrends Publishing, 2003, 206

34. National Nutritional Conference for Defense May 14, Federal Sea Agency, pp 176

35.   Family Practice News, Sept 1, 1981

36.   Schmid R. 229

37.   Krauss, W.E., Erb, J.H. and Washburn, R.G. Studies on the
       nutritive value of milk, II. The effect of pasteurization on some
       of the nutritive properties of milk," Ohio Agricultural
       Experiment Station Bulletin 518, page 9, January, 1933

38.   Schmid R 102

39.   Douglass WC. 138

40.   Howell E. 149

41.   Schmid R. 101

42.   Colpo A. The Great Cholesterol Con, Lulu, 2006, 283

43.   Rodriguez EM, Sanz AM, Diaz RC, 1999 Chemometric Studies
       of Several Minerals in Milks, Journal of Agriculture and Food
       Chemistry, 47:1520-4

44.   Consumer reports January 1974

45.   Douglass WC. 62

46.   Douglass WC. 18

47.   Annand JC. The case against milk protein. Atherosclerosis,
       1971 vol. 13, p. 137.
       Annand JC. Further evidence in the case against heated milk
       protein. Atherosclerosis, vol. 15, no. 1 (Jan. 1972), pp. 129-133.

48.   Jernigan D&S. Beating Lyme Disease: Using alternative
       medicine and god-designed living, Somerleyton Press, 2004

References

49. Hippocrates used raw milk to cure tuberculosis. Until pasteurization became the norm, medical literature extensively praised the disease-fighting ability of raw milk.
   Potter CS. Milk Diet as a Remedy for Chronic Disease, 1908

   Dr. J.E. Crewe, from the Mayo Foundation, Minnesota, reported the therapeutic uses of raw milk in 1923. For 15 years, he employed the raw-milk-diet treatment in various diseases including tuberculosis, which is ironic considering that tuberculosis was blamed on raw milk...

50. Response to letter from Ted Elkins, Deputy Director, Office of food Protection and Consumer Health Services, Maryland Department of Health and Mental Hygiene, from Sally Fallon, President, The Weston A. Price Foundation, May 23, 2006. Downloaded at www.westonaprice.org/federalupdate/aa2006/ResponseToMDH MH.pdf

51. State of Michigan Department of Community Health, PBBs (Polybrominated Biphenyls) in Michigan Frequently Asked Questions downloaded at http://www.michigan.gov/documents/mdch_PBB_FAQ_92051_ 7.pdf

   Environmental Politics and Science: The Case of PBB Contamination in Michigan MICHAEL R. REICH, PHD Am Public Health, March 1983; 73(3) 302-312

52. Brilliant LB, Wilcox K, Van Amburg G, et al: Breast-milk monitoring to measure Michigan's contamination with polybrominated biphenyls. Lancet 1978; 2:643-646

53. Schmid R.194

54. Schmid R.194-196

55. Schmid R.222, 223

56. Diez-Gonzalez F et al, Grain feeding and the dissemination of acid-resistant Escherichia coli from cattle, Science, Sept 11, 1998 281:166-168

57. Schmid R. 205

58. Douglass WC. 259, 260

59. Based on the research of Dr. Kurt Oster, summarized in Homogenized Milk May Cause Your Heart Attack - The XO Factor by Kurt A Oster. There is dispute among researchers today regarding the validity of this premise.

60. Howell E. 149

Chapter 9

61. United States Department of Agriculture Agricultural Research Magazine, August 2003 - Vol. 51, No. 8, page 18

62. Yam D, Eliraz A, Berry EM. Diet and disease--the Israeli paradox: possible dangers of a high omega-6 polyunsaturated fatty acid diet. Isr J Med Sci. 1996 Nov; 32(11): 1134-43

63. Shah PK. Plaque disruption and coronary thrombosis: new insight into pathogenesis and prevention Clin Cardiol 1997; 20(11 Suppl 2):II-38-44.

64. Colpo A, LDL Cholesterol: Bad. Cholesterol or Bad Science? Journal of American Physicians and Surgeons Volume 10 Number 3 Fall 2005

65. Felton CV, Crook D, Davies MJ, et al. Dietary polyunsaturated fatty acids and composition of human aortic plaques. Lancet 1994; 344:1195-1196.

66. Waddington E, Sienuarine K, Puddey I, Croft K Identification and quantitation of unique fatty acid oxidation products in

References

human atherosclerotic plaque using high-performance liquid chromatography. Anal Biochem. 2001 May 15; 292(2):234-44

67.   Colpo A. 57

68.   Eaton SB, Eaton SB 3rd, Sinclair AJ, Cordain L, Mann NJ Dietary intake of long-chain polyunsaturated fatty acids during the Paleolithic Period. World Rev Nutr Diet 1998; 12-23

69.   Simopoulos,A.P. 1999 Essential fatty acids in health and chronic disease. AM J Clin Nutr; 70(suppl): 560S-9S

70.   Simopoulos AP. The importance of the ratio of omega-6/omega-3 essential fatty acids. Biomed Pharmacother. 2002 Oct; 56(8):365-79

71.   McKeown P, Close Your Mouth-Buteyko Clinic handbook for perfect health, Buteyko Books, 2004, 9-13

72.   Gerster H., Can adults adequately convert alpha-linolenic acid (18:3n-3) to eicosapentaenoic acid (20:5n-3) and docosahexaenoic acid (22:6n-3)? Int J Vitam Nutr Res. 1998; 68(3):159-73

73.   Levine, Barbara S. Most Frequently Asked Questions About DHA. Nutrition Today 1997 November/December, vol. 32, pp. 248-49

74.   Gamma-Linolenic Acid By Mary G. Enig, PhD, viewed at http://www.westonaprice.org/knowyourfats/gamma-linolenic.html

75.   Enig M. Know Your Fats: The Complete Primer for Understanding the Nutrition of Fats, Oils and Cholesterol, Bethesda Press, 200, 239

76.   Sinzinger HF, Prostaglandins in the Cardiovascular System, Birkhauser Boston, 1992, pages 151-156

77.   Cambridge International Institute for Medical Science, The Scientific Calculation of the Optimum Omega6/3 Ratio, Page 24

78.   Chapkin RS, Metabolism of essential fatty acids by human epidermal enzyme preparations: evidence of chain elongation, Journal of Lipid Research, Volume 27, pages 945-954, 1986.

79.   Andersson A. et al. Fatty acid profile of skeletal muscle phospholipids in trained and untrained young men, American Journal of Endocrinological Metabolism, 279: E744-E751, 2000

80.   Shah PK. Plaque disruption and coronary thrombosis: new insight into pathogenesis and prevention Clin Cardiol 1997; 20(11 Suppl 2) :II-38-44.

81.   IBID

82.   Figures based upon Enig M. Know Your Fats, Appendix C: food Composition Tables, page 283

83.   Colpo A. 104,105

Chapter 10

84.   Stone M. 124

       Golomb BA,Criqui MH, White H,Dimsdale JE. The UCSD Statin Study: A randomized controlled trial assessing the impact of statins on noncardiac endpoints" Control Clin Trials., 2004 Apr; 25(2):178-202

       Golomb BA,Criqui MH, White H,Dimsdale JE., Conceptual Foundations of the UCSD Statin Study: A Randomized Control Trial Assessing the Impact of Statins on Cognition, Behavior, and Biochemistry") Arch Intern Med. 2004 Jan 26; 164(2):153-62.

85.   Golomb BA, McGraw J. "Lack of Physician Response Toward Perceived Statin Adverse Events" paper presented at the

References

American Heart Association, 45th Annual Conference on Cardiovascular Disease Epidemiology and Prevention in association with the Council on Nutrition, Physical Activity and Metabolism April 29–May 2, 2005, Washington D.C.

86.   Kauffman J. Myth 7 - 176

87.   NIH ClinicalTrials.gov identifier NCT00044213

88.   Fallon S. and. Enig M. Dangers of Statin Drugs: What You Haven't Been Told About Popular Cholesterol-Lowering Medicines, Viewed at http://www.westonaprice.org/moderndiseases/statin.html

89.   Kapoor R, Huang YS. Gamma linolenic acid: an antiinflammatory omega-6 fatty acid. Curr Pharm Biotechnol. 2006 Dec; 7(6):531-4.

90.   Leng GC, Lee AJ, Fowkes FG, Jepson RG, Lowe GD, Skinner ER, Mowat BF, Randomized controlled trial of gamma-linolenic acid and eicosapentaenoic acid in peripheral arterial disease.Clin Nutr. 1998 Dec; 17(6):265-71

91.   Kruger MC, Horrobin DF. Calcium metabolism, osteoporosis and essential fatty acids: a review. Prog Lipid Res .1997; 36:131-151

92.   Horrobin DF. The role of essential fatty acids and prostaglandins in the premenstrual syndrome. J Reprod Med. 1983; 28(7):465-468.

93.   Grundy SM et al, Diagnosis and Management of the Metabolic Syndrome An American Heart Association/National Heart, Lung, and Blood Institute Scientific Statement, Circulation. 2005; 112:2735-2752

94.   Nutrition Science News, July 1999, Kilmer McCully, M.D. Connects Homocysteine and Heart Disease

95.   Lahera V et al. Endothelial dysfunction, oxidative stress and inflammation in atherosclerosis: beneficial effects of statins. Curr Med Chem. 2007; 14(2):243-8

96.   Yoshida M et al, HMG-CoA reductase inhibitor modulates monocyte endothelial interaction under physiological flow condition in vitro: involvement of Rho GTPase-dependent mechanism, Arterioscler Thromb Vasc Biol. 2001; 21: 1165–1171

97.   Chopra V et al, Beyond Lipid Lowering: The Anti-Hypertensive Role of Statins., Cardiovasc Drugs Ther. 2007 Apr 28

98.   Ray KK, Lipid-independent Pleiotropic Effects of Statins in the Management of Acute Coronary Syndromes., Curr Treat Options Cardiovasc Med. 2007 Feb; 9(1):46-51

99.   Monetti M et al, Rosuvastatin displays anti-atherothrombotic and anti-inflammatory properties in apoE-deficient mice. Pharmacol Res. 2007 May; 55(5):441-9

100.   Krum H et al, Double-blind, randomized, placebo-controlled study of high-dose HMG CoA reductase inhibitor therapy on ventricular remodeling, pro-inflammatory cytokines and neurohormonal parameters in patients with chronic systolic heart failure, J Card Fail. 2007 Feb;13(1):1-7

101.   Habib A et al, Modulation of COX-2 expression by statins in human monocytic cells Faseb J. 2007 Feb 22;

102.   Shirakawa I et al. Atorvastatin attenuates transplant-associated coronary arteriosclerosis in a murine model of cardiac transplantation., Biomed Pharmacother. 2007 Feb-Apr; 61(2-3):154-9

103.   Alegret M, Silvestre JS. Pleiotropic effects of statins and related pharmacological experimental approaches. Methods Find Exp Clin Pharmacol. 2006 Nov; 28(9):627

References

104. Bruegel M, Teupser D,Haffner I,Mueller M, Thiery J. Statins reduce macrophage inflammatory protein-1alpha expression in human activated monocytes. Clin Exp Pharmacol Physiol. 2006 Dec; 33(12):1144-9.

105. Saijonmaa O, Nyman T, Fyhrquist F. Atorvastatin inhibits angiotensin-converting enzyme induction in differentiating human macrophages.. Am J Physiol Heart Circ Physiol. 2007 Apr; 292(4):H1917-21

106. Ray KK, Cannon CP, Ganz P Beyond lipid lowering: What have we learned about the benefits of statins from the acute coronary syndromes trials. Am J Cardiol. 2006 Dec 4;98(11A):18P-25P

107. Xing XQ, Gan Y, Wu SJ, Chen P, Zhou R, Xiang XD. Statins may ameliorate pulmonary hypertension via RhoA/Rho-kinase signaling pathway. Med Hypotheses. 2007;68(5):1108-13

108. Tahara N, Kai H, Ishibashi M, Nakaura H, Kaida H, Baba K, Hayabuchi N, Imaizumi T. Simvastatin attenuates plaque inflammation: evaluation by fluorodeoxyglucose positron emission tomography. Am Coll Cardiol. 2006 Nov 7;48(9):1825-31.

109. Kurumazuka D et al.Gender difference of atorvastatin's vasoprotective effect in balloon-injured rat carotid arteries. Eur J Pharmacol. 2006 Dec 28;553(1-3):263-8

110. Nagassaki S, Sertorio JT, Metzger IF, Bem AF, Rocha JB, Tanus-Santos JE. eNOS gene T-786C polymorphism modulates atorvastatin-induced increase in blood nitriteFree Radic Biol Med. 2006 Oct 1;41(7):1044-9

111. Souza-Costa DC, Sandrim VC, Lopes LF, Gerlach RF, Rego EM, Tanus-Santos JE. Anti-inflammatory effects of atorvastatin: Modulation by the T-786C polymorphism in the endothelial nitric oxide synthase gene. Atherosclerosis. 2006 Aug 26

112. Aprahamian T, Bonegio R, Rizzo J, Perlman H, Lefer DJ, Rifkin IR, Walsh K. Simvastatin treatment ameliorates autoimmune disease associated with accelerated atherosclerosis in a murine lupus model., J Immunol. 2006 Sep 1;177(5):3028-34

113. Rizzo M, Rini GB. Statins, fracture risk, and bone remodeling: What is true? Am J Med Sci. 2006 Aug ;332(2):55-60

114. Ito MK, Talbert RL, Tsimikas S. Statin-associated pleiotropy: possible beneficial effects beyond cholesterol reduction. Pharmacotherapy. 2006 Jul; 26(7 Pt 2):85S-97S

115. Hayward RA, Hofer TP, Vijan S. Narrative review: lack of evidence for recommended low-density lipoprotein treatment targets: a solvable problem. Ann Intern Med. 2006 Oct 3;145(7):520-30.

116. Hayward RA, Hofer TP, Vijan S. Narrative Review: Lack of Evidence for Recommended Low-Density Lipoprotein Treatment Targets: A Solvable Problem., Annals of Internal Medicine, Oct 3, 2006; 145 (7): 520-530

117. Statins and Lipid-Lowering Therapy: How Far Will the Benefits Go? Medscape Cardiology, 01/26/2004

118. Keys A., Atherosclerosis: A problem in newer public health. Journal of Mount Sinai Hospital 20, 118-139, 1953

119. Ravnskov U., 16-19

120. Rosamond w et al. Heart Disease and Stroke Statistics—2007 Update: A Report from the American Heart Association Statistics Committee and Stroke Statistics Subcommittee, Circulation 115 (5) e69-e171.

121. Zareba G. Torcetrapib and atorvastatin: a novel combination therapy for dyslipidemia., Drugs Today (Barc). 2006 Feb; 42(2):95-102.

References

122. USA TODAY Loss of heart drug is 'shocker' Robert Davis and Julie Schmit Dec. 3, 2006 http://www.usatoday.com/news/health/2006-12-03-pfizer-heart-drug_x.htm

123. Pfizer ends development of key cholesterol drug Pharmaceutical giant likely to slash staff, accelerate merger deals MSNBC News Services Dec. 4, 2006 http://www.msnbc.msn.com/id/16027217/

124. Nytimes End of Drug Trial Is a Big Loss for Pfizer December 4, 2006

125. USA TODAY Loss of heart drug is 'shocker' Robert Davis and Julie Schmit Dec. 3, 2006 http://www.usatoday.com/news/health/2006-12-03-pfizer-heart-drug_x.htm

126. Kastelein JJ, van Leuven SI, Burgess L, Evans GW, Kuivenhoven JA, Barter PJ, Revkin JH, Grobbee DE, Riley WA, Shear CL, Duggan WT, Bots ML; RADIANCE 1 Investigators. Effect of torcetrapib on carotid atherosclerosis in familial hypercholesterolemia. N Engl J Med. 2007 Apr 19;356(16):1620-30

127. Nissen SE, Tardif JC, Nicholls SJ, Revkin JH, Shear CL, Duggan WT,Ruzyllo W, Bachinsky WB,Lasala GP, Tuzcu EM; ILLUSTRATE Investigators. Effect of torcetrapib on the progression of coronary atherosclerosis. N Engl J Med. 2007 Mar 29;356(13):1304-16.

128. Kauffmann JM. 166

129. Late thrombosis in drug-eluting coronary stents after discontinuation of antiplatelet therapy. The Lancet, 2004 Oct 23-29;364(9444):1519-21. E. McFadden, E. Stabile, E. Regar, E. Cheneau, A. Ong, T. Kinnaird, W. Suddath, N. Weissman, R. Torguson, K. Kent

130. Boston Scientific Acknowledges Risks Tied to Stent, Wall street journal, Sylvia Pagan Westphal and Ron Winslow,September 7, 2006; Page A3

131. Camenzind E. Safety of drug-eluting stents: A meta-analysis of first generation drug-eluting stent programs.

Nordmann A. Safety of drug-eluting stents: Insights from a meta-analysis – see also:

Nordmann AJ, Briel M, Bucher HC Mortality in randomized controlled trials comparing drug-eluting vs. bare metal stents in coronary artery disease: a meta-analysis.. Eur Heart J. 2006 Dec; 27(23):2784-814

132. Boden WE, et al. Optimal medical therapy with or without PCI for stable coronary disease, N Engl J Med. 2007 Apr 12;356(15):1503-16

133. "Stent Thrombosis After Implantation of Drug Eluting Stent and Bare Metal Coronary Stents in Western Denmark", Dr. Michael Maeng, presented at the March 2007 American College of Cardiology Convention

134. Camenzind EN. Treatment of in-stent restenosis--back to the future? Engl J Med. 2006 Nov 16;355(20):2149-51

135. Lange H, et al, Folate therapy and in-stent restenosis after coronary stenting. N Engl J Med. 2004 Jun 24;350(26):2673-81.

136. Nishida T, Shimokawa H, Oi K, Tatewaki H, Uwatoku T, Abe K, Matsumoto Y, Kajihara N, Eto M, Matsuda T, Yasui H, Takeshita A, Sunagawa K. Extracorporeal cardiac shock wave therapy markedly ameliorates ischemia-induced myocardial dysfunction in pigs in vivo Circulation. 2004 ;110:3055-3061

137. Gutersohn A, Caspari G, Erbel R, Short and Long Term clinical improvement in patients with refractory angina using cardiac

shock wave therapy., Presented at the International Academy of Cardiology, 12th world Congress on Heart Disease, Vancouver, B.C. Canada July 16-19,2005

138. Fukumoto Y, Shimokawa H,et al, Extracorporeal cardiac shock wave therapy ameliorates myocardial ischemia in patients with severe coronary artery disease. Coron Artery Dis. 2006 Feb; 17(1):63-70.

139. New York Times, Lessons of Heart Disease, Learned and Ignored, April 8, 2007

140. Caspi O, Lesman A, Basevitch Y, Gepstein A, Arbel G, Habib IH, Gepstein L, Levenberg S. Tissue engineering of vascularized cardiac muscle from human embryonic stem cells., Circ Res. 2007 Feb 2;100(2):263-72.

Chapter 11

141. Flavius Josephus Contra Apionem, I, (Against Apion book 1)

142. Bishop of Bristol Robert Gray, The Connection Between the Sacred Writings and the Literature of Jewish and Heathen Authors Sec Ed, 1819 page 69

143. Schenck SE, The Live Food Factor: A comprehensive guide to the ultimate diet for body, mind spirit & planet, 1st Impression Publishing, 2006, 177

The Connection Between the Sacred Writings and the Literature of Jewish and Heathen Authors: By Bishop of Bristol Robert Gray, page 70

144. Schenck SE, 177

145. Food Science for All and a New Sunlight Theory of Nutrition – Lectures to Teachers of Domestic Economy, M. Bircher-Benner, Fourth Lecture, page 51, Republished 1960 by Health Research

146. Hans Fischer, The Nobel Prize in Chemistry 1930, Nobel Lecture, On haemin and the relationships between haemin and chlorophyll, December 11,1930

147. Hughes JH, Latner AL. Chlorophyll and haemoglobin regeneration after haemorrhage. J Physiol. 1936 May 4;86(4):388-395

148. Meyerowitz S. Power Juices, Super Drinks: Quick, Delicious Recipes to Prevent & Reverse Disease Kensington, 2000, page 92

149. Fox C, Ramsoomair D, Carter C., Magnesium: its proven and potential clinical significance. South Med J. 2001 Dec;94(12):1195-201

150. Shechter M, Bairey Merz CN, Stuehlinger HG, Slany J, Pachinger O, Rabinowitz B., Effects of oral magnesium therapy on exercise tolerance, exercise-induced chest pain, and quality of life in patients with coronary artery disease. Am J Cardiol. 2003 Mar 1;91(5):517-21

151. Wigmore A. The Wheatgrass Book: How to Grow and Use Wheatgrass to Maximize Your Health and Vitality, Avery 1985, 10,11,18,21,29,36,44, 46,34,47, 48, 59, 61, 83

152. Wigmore A., 21,34,36,47,48,59,61

    Meyerwitz S. Wheatgrass Nature's Finest Medicine: The Complete Guide to Using Grasses to Revitalize Your Health Book Publishing Company, 1999, 63,69

153. Rudolph T. Chlorophyll Nature's Green Magic, Nutritional Research, 1957

154. Jensen B. Dr. Jensen's Juicing Therapy,: Nature's Way to Better Health and a Longer Life, McGraw-Hill, 2000, 56

155. Meyerwitz S. 132

References

156. Wigmore A. 105-106

   Fallon S. 615

157. Boutenko V. Green for Life, Raw Family Publishing, 2005, 12, 16, 17, 41, 49, 50

158. Derek E. Wildman, et al. "Implications of Natural Selection in Shaping 99.4% Nonsynonomous DNA Identity Between Humans and Chimpanzees: Enlarging Genus Homo." Proceedings of the National Academy of Sciences. May 19,2003 (#2172)

159. Pilbeam D. Genetic and morphological records of the Hominoidea and hominid origins: a synthesis. Mol Phylogenet Evol. 1996 Feb;5(1):155-68

160. Harding R, Teleki G. Omnivorous Primates: Gathering and Hunting in Human Evolution, Columbia Univ. Press, 1981, 303-343

161. Scientific American, July 2001, Sigma Chi Chimpy, Forget The Ladies--For Chimps, Hunting Is About Fraternity By Meredith F. Small

162. American heart Disease website: http://www.americanheart.org/presenter.jhtml?identifier=4574

Chapter 12

163. As of this writing, on display at the University of Pennsylvania Museum of Archaeology and Anthropology

164. Health and Nutritional Properties of Probiotics in Food including Powder Milk with Live Lactic Food and Agriculture Organization of the United Nations World Health Organization, October 2001

165. Mann,G.V.1977.Hypocholesterolemic effect of milk. Lancet
      10:556

      Howard, A.N., and J. Marks. 1977. Hypocholesterolemic effect
      of milk. Lancet 30:255.

      Mann, G. V. 1977. A factor in yogurt which lowers cholesterol
      in man. Atherosclerosis 26:335.

166. Based on the research of Dr. Kurt Oster, summarized in
      Homogenized Milk May Cause Your Heart Attack - The XO
      Factor by Kurt A Oster. There is dispute among researchers
      today regarding the validity of this premise.

167. Gilbère G. Nature's Prescription Milk, Freedom Press, 2002, 27

168. Belanger J Raising Dairy Goats: Breeds, Care, Dairying. Storey
      Publishing, 2000, 122

169. Gilbère G. 28

170. US Food And Drug Administration Center for Veterinary
      Medicine, May/June 2000 FDA Veterinarian Newsletter

171. Douglass WC. 62

172. Sally Fallon and Mary G. Enig, PhD. The Ploy of Soy, Price-
      Pottinger Nutrition Foundation, San Diego, CA

173. Gilbère G. 26

174. IBID

175. Rodriguez EM, Sanz AM, Diaz RC, 1999 Chemometric Studies
      of Several Minerals in Milks, Journal of Agriculture and Food
      Chemistry, 47: 1520-4

176. Jernigan D&S. 273

References

177.   Gilbère G. 27

178.   Fomon SJ. Infant Nutrition Sec ed, W B Saunders Co. 1974, 206

179.   Maugh, T.H. Milk may be the carrier of Crohn's. The Advocate, ES, December 5, 2000.

Maugh TH II. Milk may be the carrier of Crohn's. Los Angeles Times 2000 Sep 18:S1.

180.   Stockton S. The Terrain Is Everything, Power of One Publishing, 2000, 207-208

181.   Fallon S. 87

182.   The Milwaukee Journal Sentinel, Apr 17, 2007, Whey's price going way up; Increase should be benefit for state, by Rick Barrett

183.   Vasey C. The Whey Prescription The Healing Miracle in Milk, Healing Arts Press, 2006, Chap 1 The history of Whey

184.   Fallon S. 89

185.   Fallon S. 92

186.   Townsend Letter for Doctors and Patients, July, 2003, Consuming whole foods in their raw, uncooked state: a personal interview with raw food nutrition expert, David Wolfe - Medicinal Properties in Whole Foods – Interview, Gina L. Nick

187.   Kroeger H. 64

Chapter 13

188.   Plain Language About Shiftwork, Rosa R, Colligan M, U.S. Department of Health and Human Services, Public Health

Service, Centers for Disease Control and Prevention, National Institute for Occupational Safety and Health, July 1997

189. Daytime cardiac autonomic activity during one week of continuous night shift., Fletcher A, Dorrian J, Roach G, Dawson D., J Hum Ergol (Tokyo). 2001 Dec; 30(1-2):223-8.

190. Nedley N. Proof Positive: How to Reliably Combat Disease and Achieve Optimal Health Through Nutrition and Lifestyle, Nedley Publishing 1999, Chapter 9

191. Manchester LC, Tan DX, Reiter RJ, Park W, Monist K,Qi W., High levels of melatonin in the seeds of edible plants: possible function in germ tissue protection., Life Sci. 2000 Nov 10;67(25):3023-9

192. Reiter RJ, Manchester LC, Tan DX. Melatonin in walnuts: influence on levels of melatonin and total antioxidant capacity of blood. Nutrition. 2005 Sep; 21(9):920-4

193. Colpo A. 164

194. Lee CO, Complementary and alternative medicines patients are talking about: melatonin.,Clin J Oncol Nurs. 2006 Feb;10(1):105-7

195. Nedley N. 68

196. Chen CY, Milbury PE, Lapsley K, Blumberg JB. Flavonoids from almond skins are bioavailable and act synergistically with vitamins C and E to enhance hamster and human LDL resistance to oxidation. J Nutr. 2005 Jun; 135(6):1366-73

197. Hanna Kroeger H. 64

198. Schmid 100

199. Colpo A. 126

References

200. Kritchevsky D., Cholesterol vehicle in experimental atherosclerosis. A brief review with special reference to peanut oil. Arch Pathol Lab Med. 1988 Oct; 112(10):1041-4

201. Fallon S. 563 513

Chapter 14

202. Stone M. 184

203. Grisanti R. How to Really Lose Weight After 40, third edition, ebook, Busatti Corporation, 2006 Chapter(s) 12

204. Meyer, et al. Interval vs. continuous exercise training after coronary bypass surgery: A comparison of training-induced acute reactions with respect to the effectiveness of the exercise methods. Clin Cardiol. Dec, 1990 :851-61.

205. Inbar O, Skinner JS, Bar-Or O. The Wingate Anaerobic Test, Human Kinetics, 1996, 1

206. Lunde, et al Skeletal muscle fatigue in normal subjects and heart failure patients. Is there a common mechanism? Acta Physiol Scand. 1998.

207. Lee IM, Sesso HD, Oguma Y, Paffenbarger RS Jr. Relative intensity of physical activity and risk of coronary heart disease. Circulation. 2003 Mar 4;107(8):1110-6.

208. MacDougall et al. Muscle performance and enzymatic adaptations to sprint interval training. J Appl Physiol. June, 1998

209. Burgomaster, et al. Six sessions of sprint interval training increases muscle oxidative potential and cycle endurance capacity in humans. J Appl Physiol. Feb, 2005

210. Rugnmo, et al. High intensity aerobic interval exercise is superior to moderate intensity exercise for increasing aerobic

capacity in patients with coronary artery disease. Eur J
Cardiovasc Prev Rehabil. June, 2004.

211. Parra J,Cadefau JA, Rodas G,Amigo N,Cusso R. The
distribution of rest periods affects performance and adaptations
of energy metabolism induced by high-intensity training in
human muscle. Acta Physiol Scand. 2000 Jun; 169(2):157-65.

212. IBID

213. Robergs R.A, Landwehr R. The surprising history of the
"HRmax=220-age" Equation. Journal of Exercise Physiology
Official Journal of The American Society of Exercise
Physiologists (ASEP) Volume 5 Number 2 May 2002

214. Kauffmann JM. 155 -160

215. Indoor Air Quality (IAQ), U.S. EPA and the U.S. Consumer
Product Safety Commission, Office of Radiation and Indoor Air
(6609J) EPA Document # 402-K-93-007, April 1995

216. New York Times December 24, 1972. Charles Atlas, 79, dies;
Body-Building Pioneer

217. Helgerud J, Høydal K, Wang E, Karlsen T, Berg P, Bjerkaas M,
Simonsen T, Helgesen C, Hjorth N, Bach R, Hoff J.,Aerobic
high-intensity intervals improve VO2max more than moderate
training. Med Sci Sports Exerc. 2007 Apr; 39(4):665-71

Chapter 15

218. Heil M, Eitenmuller I, Schmitz-Rixen T, Schaper W. J.
Arteriogenesis versus angiogenesis: similarities and differences.
Cell Mol Med. 2006 Jan-Mar; 10(1):45-55.

219. Tex Heart Inst J. 2004; 31(1): 47–60

References

220. Keith Brewer K. The High pH Therapy for Cancer Tests on Mice and Humans. Pharmacology Biochemistry & Behavior, v. 21, Suppl., 1, pp 1-5

221. Safian RD, Mark S. Freed MS, Cindy Grines C, The Manual of Interventional Cardiology, Physician's Press, 2001, 292

222 Safian RD, Mark S. Freed MS, Cindy Grines C, The Manual of Interventional Cardiology, Physician's Press, 2001, 287

223. Chronic Total Occlusions, Ron Waksman (Editor), Shigeru Saito (Editor), Blackwell Publishing, page 8

224. Flowcardia Inc, the manufacturer of the Crosser® CTO Recanalization Catheter http://www.flowcardia.com/patient_cto.htm – viewed Mar 1, 2010 .

225 Chronic Total Occlusions, Ron Waksman (Editor), Shigeru Saito (Editor), Blackwell Publishing, page 104, Re-entry Technique – Pioneer Catheter, Nicolaus Reifart,

226. King SB, et al. A randomized trial comparing coronary angioplasty with coronary bypass surgery. Emory Angioplasty versus Surgery Trial (EAST). N Engl J Med 1994;331(16):1011-1050

227. Dr. Clyde Yancy, president of the American Heart Association, reported by Cristian Salazar and Maryilynn Marchione, Associated Press Writers Feb 12,2010.

228. Dr. Raj Makkar, director of interventional cardiology and the cardiac catheterization laboratory at Cedars-Sinai Medical Center in Los Angeles, reported in New York Times Feb 11 ,2010

Chapter 17

229. Ravnskov U. 207

230. Colpo A. 62-64

Chapter 18

231. Time Magazine Letters to the Editor Monday, May. 12, 1980

232. University of Maryland Medical Center web site
http://www.umm.edu/altmed/articles/turmeric-000277.htm
viewed Feb 19, 2010

233. Verma SK, Bordia A, Jain P, Srivastava KC, Antioxidant
property of ginger in patients with coronary artery disease,
South Asian J Prevent. Cardiol.,Volume 8 Number 4, October -
December 2004

234. Yance D, Valentie A, Herbal Medicine, Healing & Cancer,
McGraw-Hill , 1999, 218

235 Colpo A. The Great Cholesterol Con sec edition- ebook page 289

236. Enig M. 105,106

237. Enig M. 128, 129, 250

238. Enig M. 197

239. Manku MS, Morse-Fisher N, Horrobin DF. Changes in human
plasma essential fatty acid levels as a result of administration of
linoleic acid and gamma-linolenic acid. Eur J Clin Nutr. 1988
Jan; 42(1):55-60

240. Barre DE, Holub BJ., Chapkin R.S. The effect of borage oil
supplementation on platelet aggregation, thromboxane B_2,
prostaglandin E_1 and E_2 formation. Nutr. Res. 1993; 13:739-751

241. Keen CL, Holt RR, Oteiza PI, Fraga CG, Schmitz HH, Cocoa
antioxidants and cardiovascular health, Am J Clin Nutr. 2005
Jan;81(1 Suppl):298S-303S

References

Vita JA, Polyphenols and cardiovascular disease: effects on endothelial and platelet function, Am J Clin Nutr. 2005 Jan;81(1 Suppl):292S-297S

242. Gerster H, The use of n-3 PUFAs (fish oil) in enteral nutrition. Int J Vitam Nutr Res. 1995; 65(1):3-20.

243. Fallon S. 113

244. Fallon S. 25

245. Vasey C, The Acid-Alkaline Diet for Optimum Health: Restore Your Health by Creating Balance in Your Diet, Healing Arts Press 2004, 53

246. Schmid R. 100

247. Vasey C, 55

248. Colpo A. (first ed) 62-64

249. Groschel K, Ernemann U, Schulz JB, Nagele T, Terborg, Kastrup A. Stain therapy at carotid angioplasty and stent placement: effect on procedure-related stroke, myocardial infarction, and death. Radiology. 2006 Jul; 240(1):145-51

250. Langsjoen PH. The clinical use of HMG CoA-reductase inhibitors (statins) and the associated depletion of the essential co-factor coenzymeQ_{10}; a review of pertinent human and animal data. http://www.fda.gov/ohrms/dockets/dailys/02/May02/052902/02 p-0244-cp00001-02-Exhibit_A-vol1.pdf

251. Moosmann B, Behl C. Selenoprotein synthesis and side-effects of statins., Lancet. 2004 Mar 13;363`(9412):892-4

252. Matthias Heil, Wolfgang Schaper. Influence of Mechanical, Cellular, and Molecular Factors on Collateral Artery Growth (Arteriogenesis),Circulation Research. 2004 ;95:449.

253. Heil M, Eitenmuller I, Schmitz-Rixen T,Schaper W. J. Arteriogenesis versus angiogenesis: similarities and differences. Cell Mol Med. 2006 Jan-Mar; 10(1):45-55.

254. Schaper W; Scholz D. Factors Regulating Arteriogenesis. Arteriosclerosis, Thrombosis, and Vascular Biology. 2003;23:1143

255. Schaper W, Buschmann I., Arteriogenesis,the good and bad of it, European Heart Journal (1999)20,1297–1299

256. Heil M, Eitenmuller I, Schmitz-Rixen T,Schaper W. Arteriogenesis versus angiogenesis: similarities and differences. J Cell Mol Med. 2006 Jan-Mar; 10(1):45-55.

257. Heil M, Schaper W. Influence of Mechanical, Cellular, and Molecular Factors on Collateral Artery Growth (Arteriogenesis), Circulation Research. 2004; 95:449

258. Summarized from: Buschmann I, Schaper W, Arteriogenesis Versus Angiogenesis: Two Mechanisms of Vessel Growth News Physiol Sci. 1999 Jun; 14:121-125.

259. Weis M, Heeschen C, Glassford AJ, Cooke JP. Statins have biphasic effects on angiogenesis. Circulation. 2002 Feb 12;105(6):739-45

Skaletz-Rorowski A,Walsh K. Statin therapy and angiogenesis. Curr Opin Lipidol. 2003 Dec; 14(6):599-603

References

Urbich C,, Dernbach E, Andreas M. Zeiher AM, Dimmeler S. Double-Edged Role of Statins in Angiogenesis Signaling, *Circ. Res.* 2002; 90;737-744

260. Available online
http://www.nci.nih.gov/cancertopics/understandingcancer/angio genesis/allpages and
http://www.cancer.gov/cancertopics/understandingcancer/angio genesis
(accessed March 25, 2007)

    see also Tumor angiogenesis and accessibility: role of vascular endothelial growth factor., Jain RK., : Semin Oncol. 2002 Dec; 29(6 Suppl 16):3-9

261. Folkman J. Tumor angiogenesis: therapeutic implications. N Engl J Med. 1971 Nov 18;285(21):1182-6.

262. Ferrara N. Role of vascular endothelial growth factor in physiologic and pathologic angiogenesis: therapeutic implications. Semin Oncol. 2002 Dec; 29(6 Suppl 16):10-4

263. Newman TB, Hulley SB. Carcinogenicity of lipid-lowering drugs. JAMA 1996; 275: 55-60

264. Duncan RE, El-Sohemy A, Archer MC. Statins and Cancer Development, Cancer Epidemiology Biomarkers & Prevention Vol. 14, 1897-1898, August 2005

265. Fallon S, Enig M. The Dangers of Statin Drugs- What you haven't been told about cholesterol-lowering medicines. Viewed at http://www.westonaprice.org/moderndiseases/statin.html

266. Arbiser JL, Klauber N, Rohan R, et al. Curcumin is an in vivo inhibitor of angiogenesis. Mol Med. 1998;4(6):376-383.

267. Alber HF, et al. Effect of atorvastatin on peripheral endothelial function and systemic inflammatory markers in patients with

stable coronary artery disease. Wien Med Wochenschr. 2007 Feb; 157(3-4):73-78

O'Driscoll G, Green D, Taylor RR. Simvastatin, an HMG-coenzyme A reductase inhibitor, improves endothelial function within 1 month. Circulation. 1997 Mar 4;95(5):1126-31.

268. Taneva E, Borucki K, Wiens L, Makarova R,Schmidt-Lucke C, Luley C, Westphal S. Early effects on endothelial function of atorvastatin 40 mg twice daily and its withdrawal, Am J Cardiol. 2006 Apr 1;97(7):1002-6.

269. Matsunaga T, Warltier DC, Weihrauch DW, Moniz M, Tessmer J, Chilian WM. Ischemia-Induced Coronary Collateral Growth Is Dependent on Vascular Endothelial Growth Factor and Nitric Oxide, Circulation. 2000; 102:3098

270. Ii M, Losordo DW. Statins and the endothelium. Vascul Pharmacol. 2007 Jan; 46(1):1-9.

271. Stefanie Dimmeler, et al. HMG-CoA reductase inhibitors (statins) increase endothelial progenitor cells via the PI 3-kinase/Akt pathway J Clin Invest. 2001 August 1; 108(3): 391–397.
      Llevadot J et al, HMG-CoA reductase inhibitor mobilizes bone marrow–derived endothelial progenitor cells J Clin Invest. 2001 August 1; 108(3): 399–405

      Vasa M, Fichtlscherer S, Adler K, Aicher A, Martin H,. Zeiher AM, Dimmeler S. Increase in Circulating Endothelial Progenitor Cells by Statin Therapy in Patients With Stable Coronary Artery Disease *Circulation.* 2001; 103:2885

272. Pourati, Isaac et al. Statin Use Is Associated with Enhanced Collateralization of Severely Diseased Coronary Arteries. American Heart Journal, November 2003, Volume 146, Number 5, Pages 876-881.

References

273. Dincer I, Ongun A, Turhan S, Ozdol C, Kumbasar D, Erol C. Association between the dosage and duration of statin treatment with coronary collateral development. Coron Artery Dis. 2006 Sep;17(6):561-5

274. Forte A, Cipollaro M, Cascino A, Galderisi U. Pathophysiology of stem cells in restenosis. Histol Histopathol. 2007 May; 22(5):547-57

275. Wahl P, Bloch W, Schmidt A. Exercise has a Positive Effect on Endothelial Progenitor Cells, which Could be Necessary for Vascular Adaptation Processes Int J Sports Med: DOI: 10.1055/s-2006-924364

276. Heil M, Schaper W. Insights into pathways of arteriogenesis. Curr Pharm Biotechnol. 2007 Feb;8(1):35-42

277. Schaper W. Scholz D. Factors Regulating Arteriogenesis, Arteriosclerosis, Thrombosis, and Vascular Biology. 2003 ;23:1143.

278. Colpo A. 166, 167

279. Prior BM, Lloyd PG, Ren J, Li Z, Yang HT, Laughlin MH, Terjung RL Arteriogenesis: role of nitric oxide., Endothelium. 2003; 10(4-5):207-16.

280. CNN News - Sharon heart operation set for Thursday Sunday, January 1, 2006

281. Law MR, Wald NJ, Rudnicka AR, Quantifying effect of statins on low density lipoprotein cholesterol, ischaemic heart disease, and stroke: systematic review and meta-analysis.BMJ. 2003 Jun 28;326(7404):1423

282. Heil M, Schaper W, Influence of Mechanical, Cellular, and Molecular Factors on Collateral Artery Growth (Arteriogenesis) Circulation Research. 2004; 95:449.

283. IBID

Tuttle JE et al. VZ Shear level influences resistance artery remodeling:wall dimensions,cell density,and eNOS expression. *Am J Physiol Heart Circ Physiol* 281:H1380–H1389,2001

284. Laufs U, et al. Running exercise of different duration and intensity: effect on endothelial progenitor cells in healthy subjects. Eur J Cardiovasc Prev Rehabil. 2005 Aug; 12(4):407-14

285. Hill JM,Zalos G,Halcox JP, Schenke WH, Waclawiw MA, Quyyumi AA, Finkel T. Circulating endothelial progenitor cells, vascular function, and cardiovascular risk..N Engl J Med. 2003 Feb 13;348(7):593-600

    Werner N. Circulating endothelial progenitor cells and cardiovascular outcomes. N Engl J Med. 2005 Sep 8;353(10):999-1007

286. Parra J,Cadefau JA, Rodas G,Amigo N,Cusso R. The distribution of rest periods affects performance and adaptations of energy metabolism induced by high-intensity training in human muscle. Acta Physiol Scand. 2000 Jun; 169(2):157-65.

    Grisanti R. How to REALLY Lose Weight After 40 Sec edition – ebook, 2005, chapter 12

287. Colpo A. 103

288. Batmanghelidj,F, Your Body's Many Cries for Water, Global Health   Solutions, 2004, 160-162

    Stone M. 132-135, 138

Chapter 19

289. UN General Assembly- in December 1948 and came into effect in January 1951

References

290. Nytimes December 4, 2006 End of Drug Trial Is a Big Loss for Pfizer

291. American Heart Association, 2007 update at-a-glance- Our guide to current statistics and the supplement to our "Heart and Stroke Facts" Update: Chapter 2 e73

292. Centers for Disease Control and Prevention, National Center for Health Statistics, Leading Causes of Death, 1900-1998, 67

293. Id at 44

294. C.G. Grulee et al, Breast and Artificial Feeding, Journal of the American Medical Association Sept 1934, 103(10):735

295. Douglass WC. 157

296. Id at 155, 158

297. Id at 152

Chapter 20

298. Fuster V et al. 7

Chapter 21

299 Golomb BA, Kane T, Dimsdale JE. Severe irritability associated with statin cholesterol-lowering drugs. QJM. 2004 Apr;97(4):229-35

About the author

Mike Stone grew up in Baltimore, Maryland and graduated from the University of Maryland with a bachelor's degree in Business and Public Administration. He immigrated to Israel in 1975.

In the early 80's Mike made a career change with a practical engineering degree in computer programming. After a long stint as senior systems analyst and programmer at Israel Military Industries, he made the transition to the emerging Internet field, and for eight years served as the site webmaster of a major governmental website.

Married for over 20 years, Mike and Esty live on the outskirts of Jerusalem with their four kids, Lambchop (family dog), Nivi (the cat), and a whole bunch of Nivi's relatives and friends who pop over at snack time................

Chronic Total Occlusion (previously *The Next 20,000*) is the sequel to *Surviving a Successful Heart Attack* first published in 2004.

Mike Stone survived his heart attack with flying colors, but surviving the statins was a different matter altogether. This is his story -- why he discontinued taking the statins and what convinced him that it was NOT the cholesterol that caused his heart attack. Anyone who has had a heart attack or fears one in the future will want to read Mike's harrowing experience in post heart attack life and his own conclusions (contradicting many of today's accepted cardiological doctrines) as to what really caused his own heart attack

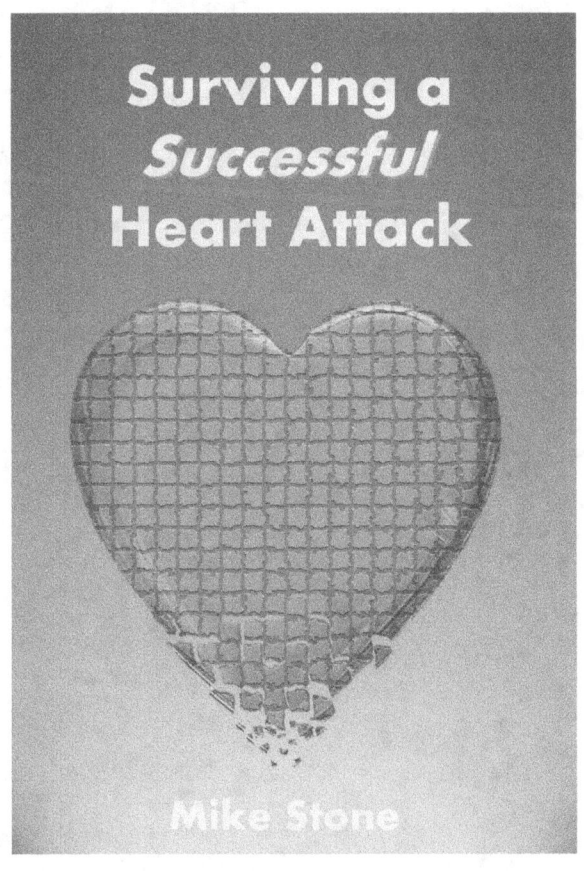